DR. BRENNAN'S DIET MENUS

Dr. Richard O. Brennan

Harvest House Publishers
Irvine, California 92714

DR. BRENNAN'S DIET MENUS

Copyright © 1978 by Richard O. Brennan

Revised Edition
Published by Harvest House Publishers
Irvine, California 92714

Library of Congress Catalog Card Number 79-91110
ISBN 0-89081-218-7

All rights reserved. No portion of this book may be reproduced in any form without the written permission of the Publisher.

Printed in the United States of America.

Contents

Foreword 7

Introduction 9
What the Bible Says About Diet

1. Food in Your Weigh 15
   How to shop for and prepare a month of 500-calorie menus

2. Daily Menus 23
   The doctor's guide to a 500-calorie diet of high protein, low fat, and low carbohydrates

3. Doubling Up 53
   Buying and cooking for a month of 100 calorie menus

4. Unthought-of Recipes 89
   Get the right balance of protein, fat, and carbohydrates in your low-calorie diets.

5. Slenderizing Snacks 115
   51 ways to feel like you're cheating—on 200 calories or less!

6. Your Friends 121
   How to know allowable foods and their caloric content

7. No Longer Ho Hum 127
   Add glamor while subtracting pounds whether at a party or in your own home

8. Make It Easy 139
   The shopping, reading, counting, and measuring that are musts for your diet

9. Consuming Calories 143
   How and why you burn calories

10. Why Exercise? 147
    How to get started on sensible exercises

11. The Enemy 153
    Foods to avoid and their caloric content

12. Marking Progress 169
    How to keep eat sheets and weight charts

WHAT THE BIBLE SAYS ABOUT DIET

When God created mankind, He intended for people to live long, healthy, and happy lives in an unpolluted and fruitful world (Genesis 1:28; 2:8-15). But beginning with the failure of the first two people, mankind has tended to pervert God's original intentions of long life coupled with physical, mental, and spiritual well-being. Some of mankind's errors have involved the earth itself (over-cultivation, pollution with harmful chemicals, etc.), while other errors have included people's tendencies to overindulge in unwholesome, fattening, or otherwise harmful foods and drinks.

Today as never before we are seeing the results of such careless living, and the results are not pleasant: heart disease and cancer are sweeping our nation and other Westernized nations in epidemic proportions. Unless this trend is reversed quickly, international suicide is almost upon us.

When God gave the first instructions for the proper human diet, He emphasized vegetarian foods (Genesis 1:29). We know from Leviticus 11:1-23 (compare Acts 10:9-6), in which the ceremonial restrictions were lifted) that foods from animal sources can also be nourishing when chosen wisely, but the fact remains that we as Americans eat far too much beef and pork for our own good health. Therefore such foods are given a subordinate position in the menus of this book.

We Americans also consume far too much alcohol—an overconsumption specifically warned about in the pages of the Bible (Proverbs 20:1; 23:29-32; plus other passages). A debate may rage about whether no alcohol or a little alcohol should be permitted, but to be on the safe side, alcohol-based foods and drinks are not included in the menus of this book.

Since overeating (of wholesome, not-so-wholesome, and downright harmful foods) is so widely practiced in the United States today, and since overeating contributes so heavily to obesity, high blood presure, heart disease (including heart attacks), and degenerative diseases of the internal organs (including cancer), calorie counts are provided throughout this book. It is almost impossible to reach and maintain the optimum weight for your most enjoyable health without keeping a daily calorie count.

Sometimes people tend to think that food control and other health-producing disciplines of life (such as proper exercise, also discussed in this book) are nothing but a necessary evil which is unfortunately necessary in order to become and stay healthy. However, as millions of now-healthy people will be happy to attest, becoming and staying healthy need not be a burdensome chore at all—it can be part of the joyous fullness of life that Christ talked about in John 10:10—"I have come that they might have life, and that they might have it more abundantly."

May this be your kind of life as you learn to take care of yourself properly today and every day for many happy years to come!

FOREWORD

Dr. R.O. Brennan has been my friend and my physician for many years. Actually I owe whatever professional accomplishments I have to his treatment and care, for I have had a continuing weight problem and have suffered from the malady of metabolic imbalance.

The doctor-author of this book has had a distinguished medical career. He has pioneered a branch of medicine long ignored and disclaimed by his peers. He founded and nurtured the International Academy of Preventive Medicine and the International Preventive Medicine Foundation, now recognized over much of the world. This has required innovative genius, tremendous courage, total disdain for powerful blasphemers and disclaimers, and more than a modicum of good old-fashioned Irish temper. The good doctor possesses all these attributes in generous amounts and is motivated by a relentless determination to serve humanity. The genuine affection in which he is held by a multitude of grateful patients across the country attests to his skill, dedication, integrity, and humanity, and to the tireless efforts of his questioning mind to improve understanding, expand research, and upgrade medical acuity and care while the process of education and information to the general public goes on.

Dr. Brennan has become one of the genuine authorities on the correlation between health and nutrition. He recognized long ago that the quantity of our years is much less important than the quality of life for ourselves, our families, and indeed all people everywhere.

This book has long been needed. It is really a working reference book for the serious dieter, for those of us who must learn and form proper nutritional habits. It is also meant for anyone who would prevent overweight and/or the development and control of one or more of the degenerative diseases. The writing is in lay language and easily understood. The recipes are all tested and proven.

I'm sure my copy will be dog-eared from constant use. I invite the reader to join me on the journey to happiness and success that becomes possible with feeling good and functioning at the top of one's potential. This book can start you toward that goal.

—Krin Holzhauser

Krin Holzhauser is a communications and public relations consultant. She is past National President of American Women in Radio and Television. She is also a broadcast journalist, world traveler, and motivational speaker.

INTRODUCTION

You will lose weight as well as look and feel great if you use the concise, easy-to-follow, and effective plans in DR. BRENNAN'S DIET MENUS. This is the easy way to a healthier, better-looking you. You know you are a Very Important Person, and you want to realize your potential. You can achieve all this by following the menus in this book.

As a physician interested in the chronic degenerative diseases, and especially their prevention, I have long been aware of our need to eliminate from our diets fat-depositing factors which can literally kill us. I have also been aware of a need for detailed information on WHAT and HOW we should eat to maintain a high-protein, low-fat, low-carbohydrate, low-calorie diet. Repeated requests from patients led to the compilation of this book of how-to-do-it menus and recipes.

These simple and exact menus are easy to shop for and easy to prepare. The daily 500-calorie and 1,000-calorie menus and recipes, plus the "slimming snack" suggestions, have been carefully selected and clinically tested. They work. Follow them and you can be confident that you are eating properly to achieve your goal—losing weight and looking great.

The 500 and 1000 calorie shopping list, menu, and recipes form the basis of a very precise plan flexible with 100 and 200 slimming snack suggestions.

It is easy to employ the 500 calorie plan by adding the 200 calorie mini-meal at bedtime plus the 100 calorie snack in mid-afternoon for an 800 calorie plan. The 100 calorie little meal in mid-morning can be added for a 900 calorie plan.

The 1000 calorie menu plans can form the basis for a

well-planned 1200, 1300, or 1400 caloric intake by simply using the snacks.

Medical science has established that people who are overweight and suffering from "adipose disease" (a chronic degenerative disease) are malnourished. They are suffering from a deficiency affecting the effective work of their metabolism. This means that you must give your body what it needs to operate healthfully—the right kind of food, not always less food. So I recommend that supplementary nutrients be taken to correct the deficiencies and replace what is missing in the restricted food plans.

It is also advisable to take these extra nutrients in order to protect yourself against the many chemicals present in today's food, water, and air. Clearly, these chemicals act to deplete your body's reserves of needed food elements. Also, diseases in your ancestry—chronic degenerative diseases such as diabetes, heart problems, and cancer—should alert you to a need for larger amounts of concentrated nutrients to deal with the metabolic hazards you may have inherited.

As I have pointed out in my earlier book, NUTRIGENETICS, it is important to become cell-wise in order to give your cells the nutrients they must have to function sufficiently. It is necessary to understand the whys of what I call "therapeutic augmentation of concentrated nutrients" in preference to vitamins, because you will then be giving your body ALL of the nutrients your cells need—not just a few synthetic chemicals. The chemical concoctions that make up most of the so-called vitamin products in our stores are inadequate.

You will need natural nutrient supplements for good health and proper weight correction. Some drugstores and supermarkets are now stocking these supplements, but you will find them in all health-food stores.

The 56 newly devised daily menu plans and the accompanying recipes are highly restrictive. They should be used under the supervision of your physician after he has evaluated your general health and metabolic state. Since overweight is a manifestation of many underlying disorders, your doctor can also take general measures to be used in conjunction with these dietary plans to give you a total health program.

A few words about using this book: the "slimming snack" suggestions have been a tremendous aid to those people who need between-meal and bedtime dietary support to aid the metabolism in maintaining a stable blood-sugar level. And, of course, they are great for people who like to eat between meals and who would otherwise eat the No-No's. Of course, these snack suggestions contain calories (just a few), which must be added to your menu plans, giving you a higher daily total calorie count.

So you see that it is very important to record all caloric values for all the foods and the beverages you consume daily. This will make you conscious of the necessity of staying within the recommended caloric limits. It will teach you which foods are "friends" in the allowable food section and also which foods are "enemies" and must be avoided.

A few foods from the "forbidden" food list are allowable on the 1000-calorie diet which are not permitted at all on the 500-calorie diet menus. The starred items on your forbidden list can be added to your allowable list on the 1000-calorie daily intake which are not permissible on the 500-calorie diet.

For example, an egg a day or meats not too high in fat are suitable for the higher caloric plan, and you will note that some fish and seafood can be added to the 1000-calorie diet as well as soups, vegetables, and miscellaneous foods. These are also starred, so watch for them when you are on the 1000-calorie dietary plan.

Water is a necessary nutrient and it is needed in very large amounts for the obese person. Water acts as a natural diuretic to help move out of the body the retained fluids in the overweight person. So it is necessary that you drink at least two, and preferably three, quarts of water a day. Since water has been contaminated with so many pollutants, it is wise to drink only distilled water, springwater, or tested well-water.

Another overlooked factor in securing vital nutrients for the chronically ill overweight person is the oxygen and/or air. Very few people take a deep breath during the day, so it is highly recommended that you use every hour the deep-breathing exercise described in the chapter on exercise.

To obtain the greatest benefit from the information here, you should follow each day's complete menu plan exactly as outlined, taking care to follow your own physician's recommendations and instructions also. Once accustomed to the plans, you may want to switch foods of similar values in the daily menu plans. Be sure, though, that you check their caloric listing in the "friendly" list or the "enemy" list. You may also wish to repeat various daily menus from time to time during the week to suit your taste and situation.

Be sure that you have made suitable adjustments to your shopping list. Be sure that you take your shopping list to the store with you so that there will be no question about what you have at home already and what you will need when you are preparing your meals and your snacks.

It is also useful to get a small notebook and write down exactly what you eat and when you eat it. It is good, too, to write down the circumstances under which you eat, such as: Are you nervous about some problem? Are you under tension because of some particular situation? Your notepad will serve as a constant reminder of your food consumption and help you follow your diet plan.

As you make your entries, write down your reason for wanting to lose weight. A single sentence will do, such as, "I want to stay young looking" or "I want to be a size 12 again."

Your top priorities for burning fat and losing weight

should be looking and feeling great, regaining your health and preventing the chronic degenerative diseases associated so frequently with overweight.

As you start your dietary plan, weigh your food portions on a diet scale or postal scale. The size of your food portion is very important. Soon you will be able to visually estimate your portions. When you are eating out, remember to check your servings before you start to eat. In this way you can estimate how much you should leave on your plate. With careful use of the charts in this book, you can enlarge your portion sizes and add other foods to the basic menus in order to provide well-rounded, healthful meals for your entire family. This will simplify your cooking chores in addition to helping you feel that your special diet isn't isolating you from the rest of your family.

An important part of your health is the way you see yourself, a feeling you can have of being an attractive, vibrant, vivacious person whom others admire. Therefore, you must work to cultivate a positive self-image. Visualize the person you want to be. Every morning take a few moments to relax. Take a deep breath, exhale slowly, and think of all your muscles relaxing, starting with the muscles of the eyelids, which are short and relax easily. Then, extend the relaxation downward to all the rest of your body. When you are in this relaxed, hypersuggestible state, fix in your mind's eye the person you want to look like—the person you were meant to be.

Visualize yourself walking down the street looking like a million, feeling like a million, and enjoying the envious glances of your own sex and the admiring glances of the opposite sex. Any time during the day that you have the opportunity, and are under a suitable, relaxed condition, close your eyes and visualize again this person you want to be.

Remember, this is your goal. You MUST set a goal. You must have an objective. And you must think of yourself enjoying the advantage of obtaining this goal. At night, be sure you use the same procedure that you use in the morning. Relax and think of what you have done all day to reach the goal you have projected for yourself.

Use the power of prayer. Say the prayer that you like as many times during the day as you can. Call upon the spiritual powers that have been given to you by your Creator. I recommend that my patients use the Serenity Prayer many times daily. It can help change your life because it will give you a profound philosophy and help you to use the divine power that is inherent in all our lives.

> God grant me the serenity to accept the things that I cannot change, the courage to change the things that I can, and the wisdom to know the difference.

Conscientious use of the planned menus and the accompanying recipes will give you the caloric control you must have. The slimming snacks will be invaluable. Use DR. BRENNAN'S DIET MENUS and you will lose weight, look good, and feel great!

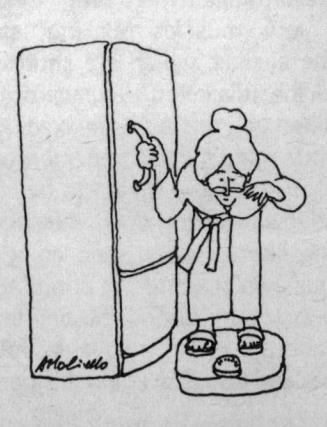

The best place for your bathroom scales is in front of your refrigerator.

1

FOOD IN YOUR WEIGH

How to shop for and prepare a month of 500-calorie menus

- Shelf control
- Complete weekly shopping lists

THE FOOD IN YOUR WEIGH

COMPLETE WEEKLY SHOPPING LISTS FOR THE 500-CALORIE PLAN, STAPLES, AND CONDIMENTS (ALL FOUR WEEKS)

Tea	Tabasco sauce
Decaffeinated coffee	Worchestershire sauce
Dietetic jelly	Chili powder
Low-calorie catsup	Caraway seed
Noncaloric sweetener	Coriander seed
Apple cider vinegar	Dry mustard
Vanilla extract	Celery salt
Lemon juice	Nutmeg
Vegetable salad oil	Black pepper
Herb seasoning	White pepper
Bay leaves	Garlic powder
Brewer's yeast	Basil
Wheat germ	Sea salt

Many years of counseling so-called "overweight" patients has forced my realization that the average American is a victim of the food industry's high-powered advertising, merchandising, and packing practices. Far too many consumers practice "impulse buying" on their food purchasing trips to the supermarket and the drive-in grocery stores.

Americans must become food-wise. They need to study labels. They must stick to the properly chosen allotted foods on their carefully planned shopping lists to insure shelf control. SHELF CONTROL means that you buy proper foods only and avoid the temptation to bring into your home any forbidden foods. Check the foods on your cabinet or refrigerator shelves, and get rid of all the forbidden foods. This will help you understand how to properly use the "foods in your weigh."

If you are eating the 100 or 200 calorie slimming snacks in addition to your daily calorie menu be sure to add the necessary food items to the shopping list. Of course, four 200 calorie snacks a day equals an 800 daily caloric intake.

Remember the best exercise is *shelf control*. Do not take anything off the grocery shelf that you should not have on the shelves in your kitchen. Should you have a weakness, it will not be available to tempt you.

For they can conquer who believe they can.

SHOPPING LISTS
500-CALORIE MENU PLAN

FIRST WEEK

MEATS & FOWL

Lean ground beef
Round steak
Beef liver
Beef franks
Turkey
Chicken liver

SEAFOODS

Fresh lobster
Fresh shrimp

BREAD PRODUCTS

Melba toast

FRUITS & BERRIES

Apple
Grapefruit
Orange
Peaches, fresh
Cantaloupe

SOUPS

Bouillon
Consomme

CHEESES & EGGS

Cottage cheese, low-fat
Egg white
Cheese, Roquefort

VEGETABLES

Asparagus, canned
String beans
Soy sprout beans
Cabbage
Cabbage, Chinese
Carrots
Celery
Chives
Cucumbers
Dandelion greens
Lettuce, iceberg
Lettuce, romaine
Okra
Onions
Onions, green
Pepper, green
Radishes
Sauerkraut, canned
Spinach
Tomato, fresh
Peas, green

BEVERAGES

Buttermilk
Skim milk
Nonfat powdered milk
Tomato juice

SECOND WEEK

MEATS & FOWL

Dried or chipped beef
Lean ground beef
Round steak
Beef liver
Bologna
Chicken fryer
Veal cutlet
Ham

BEVERAGES

Buttermilk
Skim milk
Nonfat powdered milk
Tomato juice

FRUITS & BERRIES
Apple
Cantaloupe
Lemon
Orange
Peaches, fresh
Strawberries

BREAD PRODUCTS

Melba toast
Rye-Krisp

SEAFOODS

Salmon, canned
Fresh shrimp

SOUPS

Bouillon
Consomme

CHEESES & EGGS

Cottage cheese, low-fat

VEGETABLES

Asparagus, fresh
Green beans
String beans
Soy sprout beans
Broccoli
Carrots
Celery
Lettuce, iceberg
Okra
Onions
Onions, green
Parsley
Radishes
Sauerkraut, canned
Spinach
Tomato, fresh

20
THIRD WEEK

VEGETABLES

Asparagus, fresh
Broccoli
Carrots
Celery
Cucumbers
Lettuce, iceberg
Lettuce, romaine
Mustard greens
Onions
Pepper, green
Radishes
Spinach
Tomato, fresh
Turnip greens

MEATS & FOWL

Dried or chipped beef
Lean ground beef
Beef liver
Chicken fryer
Chicken liver
Turkey
Veal cutlet
Ham

FRUITS & BERRIES

Apple
Cantaloupe
Lemon
Orange
Blueberries
Strawberries

BEVERAGES

Nonfat powdered milk
Tomato juice

SEAFOODS

Bass
Crab
Fresh shrimp
Tuna

BREAD PRODUCTS

Melba toast

CHEESES & EGGS

Cottage cheese, low-fat

SOUPS

Bouillon
Chicken

FOURTH WEEK

BEVERAGES

Buttermilk
Skim milk
Nonfat powdered milk
Tomato juice

SEAFOODS

Bass
Crab
Salmon, canned

VEGETABLES

Artichoke
Asparagus, fresh
Green beans
Cabbage
Cauliflower
Celery
Lettuce, romaine
Onions
Onions, green
Pepper, green
Tomato, fresh

BREAD PRODUCTS

Melba toast

CHEESES & EGGS

Cottage cheese, low-fat

MEATS & FOWL

Dried or chipped beef
Lean ground beef
Round steak
Sirloin
Liver (beef)
Turkey

FRUITS & BERRIES

Apple
Oranges
Peaches, fresh

SOUPS

Bouillon
Chicken

What most of us are really looking for is a diet-free diet.

To wish to be well is a part of becoming well.
—Seneca

Health and cheerfulness make beauty.
—Cervantes

They shall lay hands on the sick and they shall recover.
—Mark 16:18

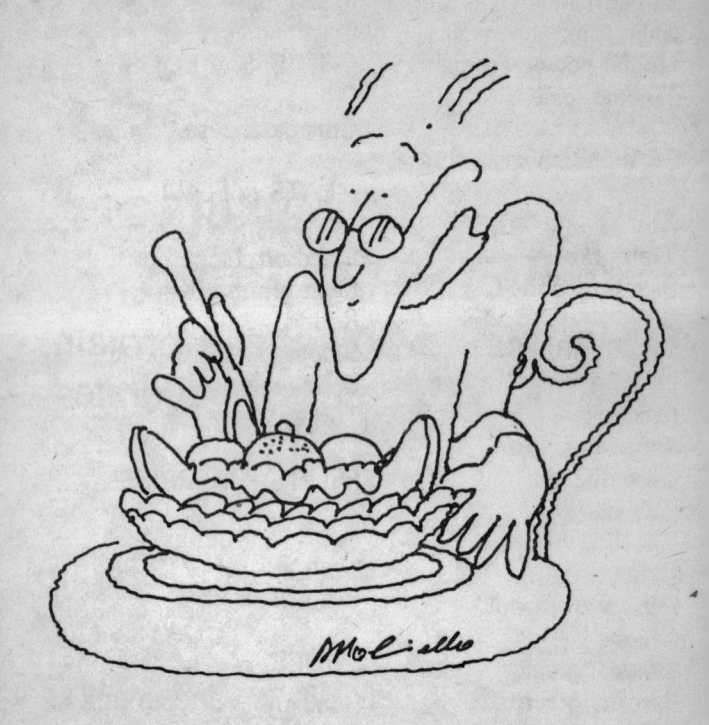

Nothing is as fattening as a spoon when you put it into a banana split.

2

DAILY MENUS
The doctor's guide to a 500-calorie diet of high protein, low fat, and low carbohydrates

- Suggested menus
- Breakfast, lunch, dinner, and snack menus for each day

MONDAY

Breakfast

½ cup nonfat cottage cheese, topped with	105
1 tsp. vegetable-type bacon	45
1 cup decaffeinated coffee	—
	150

Midmorning Snack

1 med. raw apple	80

Lunch

1 cup plain consomme, hot	30
½ large dill pickle	10
1 large slice melba toast	40
	80

Midafternoon Snack

Asparagus salad:

3 canned asparagus tips	15
2 oz. lettuce, shredded, topped with	10
sprinkle of caraway seeds	—
1 cup hot noncaloric sweetened tea	—
	25

Dinner

1 all-beef frank, grilled, drained,	110
with dash of horseradish	—
wrap in 5 large romaine lettuce leaves	10
½ cup raw carrots, sliced	25
1 round melba toast	20
Non-caloric sweetened tea, hot or cold	—
	165

Total calories for the day—500

Ye shall know the truth, and the truth shall make you free.

—John 8:32

TUESDAY

Breakfast

1 med. grapefruit, topped with	110
1 egg white, broiled	15
1 cup Bouillon, canned	30
1 large slice melba toast	40
1 cup decaffeinated coffee	—
	195

Midmorning Snack

*Celery stuffed—1 portion	15

Lunch

Green salad:

¼ cup raw spinach, shredded	10
¼ cup lettuce, shredded	5
4 med. radishes, sliced	5
½ med. tomato, sliced with herb dressing	15
1 Tbsp. apple cider vinegar	5
1 round melba toast	20
1 glass noncaloric sweetened iced tea	—
	65

Dinner

3 oz. beef liver, broiled & drained	170
½ cup string beans	15
1 large slice melba toast	40
Noncaloric sweetened tea, hot or cold	—
	225

Total calories for the day—500

WEDNESDAY

Breakfast
1½ oz. beef round steak, grilled & drained of fat	95
1 large slice melba toast	40
1 Tbsp. dietetic jelly	—
1 cup decaffeinated coffee	—
	135

Lunch
*1 serving raw vegetable mold	25
1 round melba toast	20
1 glass noncaloric sweetened tea, iced	—
	45

Dinner
*1 serving mock spaghetti with meatballs	290
3 young green onions	10
1 round melba toast	20
1 cup noncaloric sweetened, hot tea	—
	320

Total calories for the day—500

Seconds count—especially when dieting.

THURSDAY

Breakfast

½ med. cantaloupe; topped with	45
½ cup nonfat cottage cheese,	105
1 cup decaffeinated coffee	—
	150

Midmorning Snack

1 bouillon cube in 1 cup hot water	5
1 large slice melba toast	40
(may be saved for bedtime snack)	45

Lunch

*1 serving tomato aspic, served on	40
½ cup lettuce, shredded	10
1 glass hot tea, thin lemon slice	5
	55

Dinner

*1 serving tomato aspic, served on	215
4 pods cooked okra	15
1 round melba toast	20
	250

Total calories for the day—500

You are young at any age if you are making plans for tomorrow.

FRIDAY

Breakfast

1 cup bouillon, canned, hot	30
3 oz. chicken livers, broiled & drained	115
1 large slice melba toast	40
1 cup decaffeinated coffee	—
	185

Midmorning Snack

1 med. raw apple	80

Lunch

*1 serving consomme bouquetiere	25
1 round melba toast	20
1 cup hot tea, thin lemon slice	5
	50

Dinner

*1 serving cold shrimp bisque	140
½ cup sauerkraut, canned	25
½ med. raw tomato, sliced with	15
4 small radishes	5
1 glass noncaloric sweetened tea, iced	—
	185

Total calories for the day—500

Nobody may love the fat person, but many diseases are fond of them.

SATURDAY

Breakfast
½ cup raw peach, sliced with	40
½ cup nonfat cottage cheese	105
1 large slice melba toast	40
1 cup decaffeinated coffee	—
	185

Midmorning Snack
4 oz. tomato juice	30
1 round melba toast	20
	50

Lunch
½ cup canned sauerkraut	20
1 Rye-Krisp cracker	20
1 glass noncaloric sweetened tea, iced	—
	40

Dinner
*1 serving Chili-Marvel	155
1 large slice melba toast	40
1 glass noncaloric sweetened tea, hot or cold,	—
	195

Bedtime Snack
1 cup plain bouillon, served hot	30

Total calories for the day—500

Blessed is the man whose strength is in Thee.
—Psalm 84:5

SUNDAY

Breakfast
1 cup plain consomme, hot; mixed with	30
1 envelope unflavored gelatin	30
1 large slice melba toast	40
1 med. orange, sliced	80
1 cup decaffeinated coffee	—
	180

Midmorning Snack
1 stalk celery, topped with	10
2 Tbsp. nonfat cottage cheese	30
	40

Lunch
1 cup (8 oz.) tomato juice	60
1 round melba toast	20
	80

Dinner
4 oz. lobster, broiled & drained, thin lemon slice	95
1 cup Chinese cabbage	35
1 large slice melba toast	40
1 glass noncaloric sweetened tea, iced	—
	170

Bedtime Snack
1 cup bouillon, canned hot	30

Total calories for the day—500

I will restore health unto thee.

—*Jeremiah 30:17*

MONDAY

Breakfast

3 oz. lean baked ham, broiled & drained	140
1 large slice melba toast	40
1 cup decaffeinated coffee	—
	180

Midmorning Snack

1 med. apple	80

Lunch

½ cup strawberries, fresh or frozen, noncaloric sweetened, sprinkled with	30
1 envelope Knox gelatin	30
1 round melba toast	20
	80

Dinner

3 oz. fresh shrimp, boiled, topped with	70
2 Tbsp. tomato sauce	5
½ cup fresh spinach, cooked or canned, garnished with	35
1 Tbsp. raw onion, chopped	5
1 large slice melba toast	40
Noncaloric sweetened tea, hot or cold	—
	150

Bedtime Snack

1 bouillon cube in 1 cup hot water	5
1 med. celery stalk	5
	10

Total calories for the day—500

They that seek the Lord shall not lack any good thing.
—Psalm 34:10

TUESDAY

Breakfast

1 med. orange, peeled and sectioned, mixed with—	80
1 oz. dried beef, chopped	50
1 large slice melba toast	40
1 cup decaffeinated coffee	—
	170

Lunch

*1 cup clear onion soup	15
*1 serving turkey roll	30
1 Rye-Krisp cracker	20
Noncaloric sweetened tea, hot or cold	—
	65

Dinner

1 chicken thigh, fryer skin removed and broiled	150
½ cup green beans	15
½ med. raw tomato, sliced	15
1 glass (8 oz.) skim milk	85
	265

Total calories for the day—500

The secret of happiness is not in doing what one likes but in liking what one has to do.

—Barrie

WEDNESDAY

Breakfast

3 oz. lean ground beef patty, broiled	190
1 large slice melba toast topped with	40
1 peach half, water-packed or noncaloric sweetened, broiled	15
1 cup decaffeinated coffee	—
	245

Midmorning Snack

½ med. apple	40

Lunch

3 oz. fresh shrimp, boiled	70
*1 serving Tomato Aspic	40
1 Rye-Krisp cracker	20
Noncaloric sweetened tea, hot or cold	—
	130

Dinner

1 cup consomme, hot with herb seasoning	30
½ cup raw carrots, sliced	25
1 round melba toast	20
1 cup hot tea, thin lemon slice	5
	80

Bedtime Snack

1 bouillon cube in 1 cup hot water	5

Total calories for the day—500

Fear none of those things.

—Revelation 2:10

THURSDAY

Breakfast

3 oz. round steak, broiled, fat drained	190
1 large slice melba toast	40
1 cup decaffeinated coffee	—
	230

Lunch

1 med. chicken fryer thigh, (skin removed) broiled	150
*Carrot and cottage cheese salad, 1 serving	40
1 Rye-Krisp cracker	20
Noncaloric sweetened tea, hot or cold	—
	210

Dinner

½ med. cantaloupe, filled with	45
1 Tbsp. nonfat cottage cheese	15
1 cup noncaloric sweetened tea, hot	—
	60

Total calories for the day—500

Happiness lies, first of all, in Health.
—*George William Curtis*

FRIDAY

Breakfast
Breakfast cocktail; combine in blender
1 cup skim milk	85
1 Tbsp. skim milk powder	25
½ cup strawberries,	30
noncaloric sweetened to taste	—
1 large slice melba toast	40
	180

Midmorning Snack
1 peach half, water-packed or	
noncaloric sweetened, topped with	15
1 Tbsp. nonfat cottage cheese	15
1 cup decaffeinated coffee	—
	30

Lunch
3 oz. pink salmon, canned. Drain,	
break into chunks and mix with	120
½ cup fresh raw spinach, shredded	25
½ cup fresh lettuce, shredded	15
1 med. celery stalk, chopped	10
1 Tbsp. apple cider vinegar	5
Noncaloric sweetened tea, hot or cold	
	175

Dinner
1 slice all beef bologna, 4½" x 1/8"	
grill in oven, top with	70
½ cup canned sauerkraut, heated	25
1 round melba toast	20
Noncaloric sweetened tea, hot or cold	—
	115

Total calories for the day—500

SATURDAY

Breakfast

1½ oz. chipped, dried beef mixed with	80
½ cup noncaloric sweetened strawberries	30
1 large slice melba toast	40
1 cup decaffeinated coffee	—
	150

Lunch

3 oz. beef liver, broiled, fat drained	170
½ cup spinach	30
1 Rye-Krisp cracker	20
1 cup hot tea, thin slice lemon	5
	225

Dinner

3 oz. fresh shrimp, boiled, garnished with	70
1 Tbsp. raw parsley, chopped	—
½ cup broccoli, seasoned with herb seasoning	25
1 glass noncaloric sweetened tea, iced	—
	95

Bedtime Snack

1 cup plain consomme, hot	30

Total Calories for the day—500

And the Lord will take away from thee all sickness, and will put none of the evil diseases of Egypt, which thou knowest, upon thee; but will lay them upon all them that hate thee.

—Deuteronomy

SUNDAY

Breakfast

1 serving applesauce gelatin, topped with	70
2 Tbsp. vegetable-type bacon	90
1 large slice melba toast	40
1 cup decaffeinated coffee	—
	200

Lunch

*Chow mein special, 1 serving	170
½ cup green string beans	15
1 Rye-Krisp cracker	20
1 glass noncaloric sweetened tea	—
	205

Dinner

½ cup cantaloupe, 5" diam., filled with	45
2 Tbsp. nonfat cottage cheese topped with	30
Sprinkle of coriander seed	—
	75

Bedtime Snack

*Clear onion soup, 1 cup	15
1 med. celery stock	5
	20

Total calories for the day—500

*Where there is a will—
there will be less weigh.*

MONDAY

Breakfast

3 oz. lean ground beef patty broiled & drained of fat	190
1 large slice melba toast	40
1 cup decaffeinated coffee	—
	230

Midmorning Snack

1 med. orange	80

Lunch

3 oz. fresh shrimp, boiled	70
6 fresh asparagus tips, cooked, topped with	15
1 Tbsp. raw onion, chopped	5
1 glass noncaloric sweetened tea	—
	90

Midafternoon Snack

½ cup raw carrots	25

Dinner

1 cup plain bouillon, canned, topped with	30
dash of celery salt	—
1 large slice melba toast	40
	70

Bedtime Snack

1 bouillon cube in 1 cup hot water with	5
Herb seasoning	—
	5

Total calories for the day—500

He sent his word, and healed them.

—Psalm 107:20

TUESDAY

Breakfast
Filled cantaloupe:
½-5" diam. fresh cantaloupe, filled with	45
½ cup strawberries, fresh or frozen	30
¼ cup blueberries, fresh or frozen	20
2 Tbsp. nonfat cottage cheese	30
1 large slice melba toast	40
1 cup decaffeinated coffee	—
	165

Midmorning Snack
½ cup tomato juice	30
½ cup envelope unflavored gelatin	15
1 round melba toast	20
	65

Lunch
¼ med. head lettuce, shredded, topped with	20
4 radishes, chopped, with herb seasoning	5
1 round melba toast	20
1 glass noncaloric sweetened tea	—
	45

Dinner
*1 serving chow mein special	170
½ cup raw carrots, sliced	25
1 round melba toast	20
1 cup hot tea, thin slice lemon	5
	220

Bedtime Snack
1 bouillon cube in 1 cup hot water	5

Total calories for the day—500

WEDNESDAY

Breakfast
1 chicken breast, skin removed, broiled & drained	200
1 large slice melba toast	40
1 cup decaffeinated coffee	
	240

Midmorning Snack
1 cup bouillon, canned, hot	30

Lunch
3 oz. beef liver, broiled & drained	115
4 pods boiled okra	15
1 glass noncaloric sweetened tea, iced	—
	130

Dinner
Molded Salad:
1 envelope unflavored gelatin	30
1 Tbsp. lemon juice	5
¾ cup water	—
½ cup noncaloric sweetened strawberries	30
2 Tbsp. nonfat cottage cheese, served on	30
2 large romaine lettuce leaves	5
1 cup noncaloric sweetened tea, hot	—
	100

Total calories for the day—500

THURSDAY

Breakfast

3 oz. turkey, roasted	190
1 large slice melba toast	40
1 Tbsp. dietetic jelly	—
1 cup decaffeinated coffee	—
	230

Midmorning Snack

1 stalk celery	10

Lunch

4 oz. white bass, steamed, topped with	115
½ cup mustard greens, cooked	15
4 small radishes, chopped	5
1 glass noncaloric sweetened tea, iced	—
	135

Dinner

½ cup (4 oz.) clear chicken soup	40
1 med. orange	80
	120

Bedtime Snack

1 bouillon cube in 1 cup hot water	5

Total calories for the day—500

FRIDAY

Breakfast

½ cup nonfat cottage cheese, mixed with	100
½ cup strawberries, noncaloric sweetened	30
1 large slice melba toast	40
1 cup decaffeinated coffee	—
	170

Midmorning Snack

½ med. cantaloupe	45

Lunch

3 oz. chicken livers, boiled & drained	115
½ cup broccoli	25
½ med. raw cucumber, sliced	15
1 cup noncaloric sweetened tea, hot	—
	155

Dinner

Salad:

½ cup fresh raw spinach, shredded	25
½ cup fresh lettuce, shredded	15
1 Tbsp. apple cider vinegar	5
1 tsp. vegetable type bacon	45
1 large slice melba toast	40
1 glass noncaloric sweetened tea, iced	—
	130

Total calories for the day—500

SATURDAY

Breakfast

3 oz. veal cutlet, broiled & drained	175
1 large slice melba toast	40
1 Tbsp. dietetic jelly	—
1 cup decaffeinated coffee	—
	215

Midmorning Snack

1 med. apple	80

Lunch

1 bouillon cube in 1 cup hot water	5
¼ raw green pepper, sliced	5
1 large slice melba toast	40
	50

Dinner

½ med. raw tomato, cut & topped with	15
3 oz. water-packed tuna served on	130
5 large romaine lettuce leaves	
1 glass noncaloric sweetened tea, iced	—
	155

Total calories for the day—500

For they can conquer who believe they can.

SUNDAY

Breakfast

3 oz. baked ham	140
½ cup fresh strawberries, noncaloric sweetened	30
1 large slice melba toast	40
1 cup decaffeinated coffee	—
	210

Lunch

Fruit Cup:

¼ med. apple, chopped	20
¼ med. orange, chopped	20
½ med. celery stalk, chopped, served on	5
3 large romaine lettuce leaves	5
1 cup noncaloric sweetened tea, hot	5

Dinner

6 oz. crab meat, canned or fresh	170
Dash of lemon juice	5
½ cup turnip greens, boiled	25
1 large slice melba toast	40
1 cup noncaloric sweetened tea, hot or cold	—
	240

Total calories for the day—500

Health surpasses riches.

—Bailey

MONDAY

Breakfast

1 med. orange, sliced	80
*2 dried beef rolls	70
1 large slice melba toast	40
1 Tbsp. dietetic jelly	—
1 cup decaffeinated coffee	—
	190

Lunch

1 peach half, water-packed or noncaloric sweetened topped with	15
2 Tbsp. nonfat cottage cheese with nutmeg	30
	45

Dinner

*Liver beef burger, 1 serving	185
½ cup cabbage, boiled	25
1 large slice melba toast	40
Noncaloric sweetened tea, hot or cold	—
	250

Bedtime Snack

*1 cup clear onion soup, hot	15

Total calories for the day—500

From health contentment springs.
—Beattie

TUESDAY

Breakfast

4 oz. tomato juice	30
1 large slice melba toast, topped with	40
1½ oz. dried beef	80
1 cup decaffeinated coffee	—
	150

Midmorning Snack

1 celery stalk	10
1 bouillon cube in 1 cup hot water	5
	15

Lunch

3 oz. pink salmon, canned	120
½ cup green beans	15
1 large slice melba toast	40
1 glass noncaloric sweetened tea, iced	—
	175

Midafternoon Snack

½ cup raw cabbage, shredded, mixed with	15
½ med. green pepper, raw, chopped	10
	25

Dinner

1 peach half, water-packed or noncaloric sweetened, filled with	30
2 Tbsp. nonfat cottage cheese with nutmeg	
5 large romaine lettuce leaves	10
	55

Bedtime Snack

4 oz. nonfat buttermilk	40

Total calories for the day—500

WEDNESDAY

Breakfast

2 large romaine lettuce leaves topped with	5
*1 serving turkey salad	150
4 oz. tomato juice	30
1 large slice melba toast	40
1 cup decaffeinated coffee	—

Lunch

½ glass (4 oz.) skim milk	45
1 round melba toast	20
	65

Dinner

3 oz. pink salmon, canned	120
*1 cup cauliflower in sauce	55
1 slice melba toast	40
1 glass noncaloric sweetened tea, iced	—
	215

Total calories for the day—500

Overweight persons have the figures to prove that they are no good at counting calories.

Look to your health: and if you have it, praise God, and value it next to a good conscience.
—Walton

THURSDAY

Breakfast
*1 serving applesauce gelatin	70
1½ oz. dried beef	80
1 large slice melba toast	40
1 cup decaffeinated coffee	—
	190

Midmorning Snack
1 med. orange	80

Lunch
*1 serving carrot & cottage cheese salad	40
1 round melba toast	20
1 glass noncaloric sweetened tea, iced	—
	60

Dinner
*1 serving tomato baked fish	135
1 med. artichoke, steamed	15
1 round melba toast	20
1 glass tea, hot or cold	—
	170

Total calories for the day—500

The snack that you sneak . . . could be the pause that refreshes.

FRIDAY

Breakfast
3 oz. crabmeat, canned or cooked	85
1 large slice melboa toast	40
1 cup decaffeinated coffee	125

Midmorning Snack
1 med. apple	80

Lunch
½ cup clear chicken soup	40
1 round melba toast	20
1 cup noncaloric sweetened tea, hot thin slice lemon	5
	65

Dinner
2 oz. beef sirloin, grilled with	170
½ cup cooked mushrooms	25
1 cup cooked cauliflower with herb seasoning	35
Noncaloric sweetened tea, hot or cold	230

Total calories for the day—500

SATURDAY

Breakfast
*1 serving baked tomato with meat stuffing	135
1 large slice melba toast	40
1 cup decaffeinated coffee	—
	175

Midmorning Snack
*1 portion chipped beef roll	20
1 cup noncaloric sweetened tea, hot or cold	—
	20

Lunch
1 cup consomme	30
1 round melba toast	20
	50

Dinner
4 oz. white bass, steamed	115
6 fresh cooked asparagus tips, garnished with	15
1 Tbsp. raw onion, chopped	5
1 large slice melba toast	40
1 cup noncaloric sweetened tea, hot or cold	—
	175

Bedtime Snack
1 med. orange	80

Total calories for the day—500

SUNDAY

Breakfast
*2 servings turkey rolls	60
1 large slice melba toast	40
1 Tbsp. dietetic jelly	—
1 cup decaffeinated coffee	—
	100

Midmorning Snack
1 med. orange	80

Lunch
1 med. raw tomato, filled with	35
2 Tbsp. nonfat cottage cheese	30
1 young green onion	5
1 glass noncaloric sweetened tea, iced	—
	70

Dinner
*1 serving Swiss steak	225
1 round melba toast	20
1 cup noncaloric sweetened tea, hot, thin slice lemon	5
	250

Total calories for the day—500

A cheerful look makes a dish a feast.
—*Jacula Prudentum*

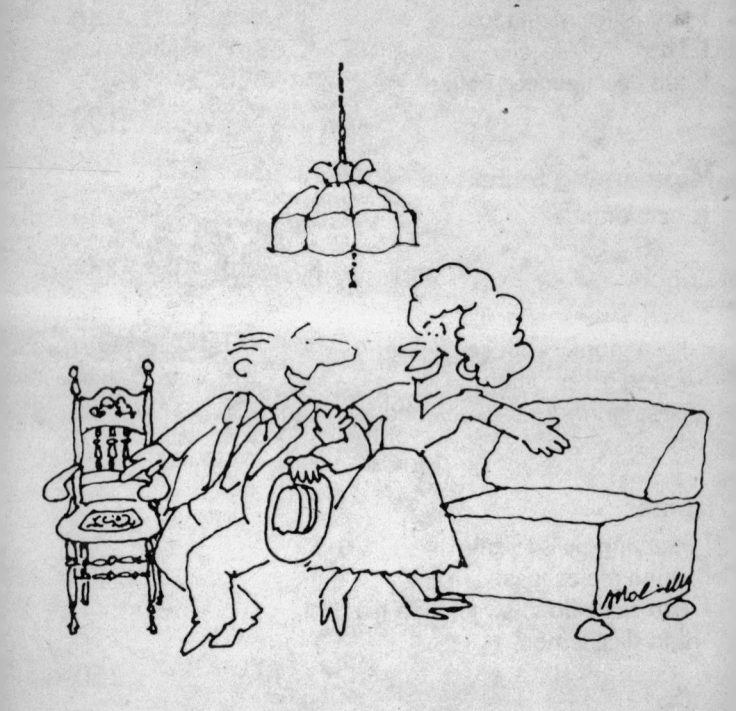

Sometimes the first time a man realizes that he's putting on weight is when the hostess begins steering him away from her antique chair.

3

DOUBLING UP
Buying and cooking
for a month of
1000-calorie menus

※

- Choosing the best calories
- Complete weekly shopping list
- Breakfast, lunch, dinner, and snack menus for each day

FOOD IN YOUR WEIGH
COMPLETE WEEKLY SHOPPING LISTS
FOR THE 1000-CALORIE PLAN

Many of these items are also on your 500-calorie shopping list. In order to avoid duplication, be sure to review the information on the 500-calorie shopping list.

STAPLES AND CONDIMENTS FOR ALL FOUR WEEKS

Bouillon cubes
Lemon extract
Dietetic margarine
Tapioca
Farina
Mint
Celery salt
Flour
Horseradish
Gelatin
Buckwheat
Paprika
Chives
Cornbread
Marjoram
Parsley
Ginger snaps
Fruit cocktail
Italian dressing
French dressing
Pickles
Yogurt
Vegetable-type bacon
Bran flakes
Sole
Tea
Decaffeinated coffee
Dietetic jelly
Noncaloric sweetener
Brewer's yeast
Wheat germ
Vinegar
Worcestershire sauce
Bay leaves
Chili sauce
Tabasco sauce
Soybean oil
Apple cider vinegar
Garlic buds
Herb seasoning
Pepper
Sea salt
Salt
Low-calorie catsup

SHOPPING LISTS
1000-CALORIE MENU PLAN

FIRST WEEK

VEGETABLES

Asparagus, fresh
Green beans
String beans
Carrots
Cauliflower
Celery
Eggplant
Lettuce, iceberg
Mushrooms
Okra
Onions, green
Radishes
Spinach
Squash, soft shell
Tomato, fresh
Blackeyed peas

MEATS & FOWL

Lean ground beef
Round steak
Tenderloin
Liver
Chicken, fryer
Turkey

SEAFOODS

Salmon, canned
Shrimp, fresh
Tuna

SOUPS

Consomme

BEVERAGES

Skim milk
Tomato juice
Vegetable juice (V-8)

BREAD PRODUCTS

Rye-Krisp
Whole wheat bread

CHEESES & EGGS

Cottage cheese, lowfat
Eggs

FRUITS & BERRIES

Apple
Cantaloupe
Grapefruit
Orange
Peaches, fresh
Strawberries
Applesauce
Pineapple
Pears

SECOND WEEK

BEVERAGES

Skim milk
Nonfat powdered milk
Tomato juice

BREAD PRODUCTS

Whole wheat bread

CHEESES & EGGS

Cottage cheese, low-fat
Eggs

FRUITS & BERRIES

Apple
Cantaloupe
Grapefruit
Lemon
Orange
Peaches, fresh
Strawberries
Salad fruits
Banana

MEATS & FOWL

Dried or chipped beef
Lean ground beef
Sirloin
Beef franks
Chicken, fryer
Veal cutlet

SEAFOODS

Shrimp, fresh
Trout

VEGETABLES

Asparagus, fresh
Beans, green
String beans
Broccoli
Cabbage
Carrots
Carrots
Cauliflower
Celery
Eggplant
Lettuce, iceberg
Onions
Onions, green
Pepper, green
Sauerkraut, canned
Squash, soft shell
Tomato, canned
Tomato, fresh

THIRD WEEK

VEGETABLES

Asparagus, fresh
Green beans
String beans
Broccoli
Cabbage
Carrots
Celery
Eggplant
Lettuce, iceberg
Mushrooms
Onions
Onions, green
Pepper, green
Squash, soft shell
Tomato, canned
Tomato, fresh

BEVERAGES

Skim milk
Tomato juice

BREAD PRODUCTS

Rye-Krisp
Whole wheat bread

CHEESES & EGGS

Cottage cheese, lowfat
Eggs

FRUITS & BERRIES

Apple
Cantaloupe
Grapefruit
Lemon
Orange
Peaches, fresh
Strawberries
Salad fruits
Pears
Banana
Cranberry sauce

MEATS & FOWL

Dried or chipped beef
Lean ground beef
Beef franks
Chicken, fryer
Chicken liver
Turkey
Veal cutlet

SEAFOODS

Shrimp, dry-packed
Shrimp, fresh
Tuna

SOUPS

Bouillon
Consomme

FOURTH WEEK

MEATS & FOWL

Lean ground beef
Sirloin
Beef franks
Chicken, fryer
Turkey

SEAFOODS

Perch
Salmon, canned
Shrimp, fresh
Trout
Flounder

BEVERAGES

Skim milk
Tomato juice
Vegetable juice (V-8)
Orange juice

BREAD PRODUCTS

Saltines
Rye-Krisp
Whole wheat bread

CHEESES & EGGS

Cottage cheese, lowfat
Eggs

FRUITS & BERRIES

Grapefruit
Lemon
Orange
Peaches, fresh
Plums, fresh
Blackberries
Strawberries
Salad fruits
Applesauce
Pineapple

VEGETABLES

Asparagus, fresh
Green beans
String beans
Cabbage
Carrots
Cauliflower
Celery
Lettuce, iceberg
Mushrooms
Okra
Onions
Onions, green
Pepper, green
Radishes
Squash, soft shell
Tomato, canned
Tomato, fresh
Green peas
Potatoes
Noodles
English peas

THE 1000-CALORIE DIET MENUS

These 1000-calorie diet menus are designed to provide a high ratio of protein and a low ratio of fats and carbohydrates. Your doctor may want you to use the 1000-calorie daily intake plan after you have been on the 500-calorie program, or you may want to start and stay on this plan according to his recommendations.

Persons who are overweight and suffering from adipose disease are malnourished. It is recommended that supplementary nutrients be taken to protect against these deficiencies and to augment those missing in your food. It is also necessary to take extra nutrients to protect against the many chemicals which are present in today's food.

Be sure that you record all the caloric values for all the food and beverages you consume. This will make you more conscious of the necessity of staying within the recommended caloric limits and teach you which foods are "friends" and which are "enemies" of good health.

A few items from the forbidden foods list are permissible on the 1000-calorie plan which are absolutely not permitted on the 500-calorie plan. An egg a day or meats not too high in fat are suitable for the higher-calorie plan. These are starred in the list.

Some fish and seafood can be added to the 1000-calorie plan, as well as soups, vegetables, and miscellaneous foods. You will find these all starred. Recipes marked with a star are found in Chapter 4, "Unthought-of-Recipes."

Dear Lord, I will fear no evil, for Thou art with me.
—Psalm 23:4

1000 CALORIES

SUNDAY

Breakfast

½ cup orange & grapefruit sections, canned, water-packed or noncaloric sweetened, mixed with	50
1½ tsp. brewer's yeast	15
3 oz. lean ground beef patty, broiled	190
1 egg, poached	75
1 slice whole wheat bread, toasted	60
1 Tbsp. dietetic jelly	—
Coffee, black	—
	390

Lunch

Shrimp salad: mix together	
3 oz. shrimp, boiled	100
½ cup celery, chopped	10
¼ head lettuce, chopped	20
½ med. tomato, sliced	20
1 Tbsp. low-calorie French dressing	5
2 crackers, saltines, 2" square	30
½ cup lowfat yogurt, mixed with	55
½ cup strawberries	30
Noncaloric tea, sweetened	—
	270

Dinner

3 oz. beef tenderloin, broiled	225
6 tips fresh asparagus, cooked	15
1 cup yellow summer squash	55
½ cup applesauce, noncaloric sweetened	45
Tea or decaffeinated coffee, black	—
	340

Total calories for the day—1000

MONDAY

Breakfast

2½ slices pineapple, water-packed or noncaloric sweetened, topped with	65
1 cup low-fat cottage cheese	205
1 slice whole wheat bread, toasted	60
Coffee, black	—
	330

Lunch

8 oz. flounder, steamed	220
Salad:	
4 oz. fresh lettuce, chopped	20
½ med. raw tomato, sliced	20
2 fresh green onions	10
½ pickle	10
2 tsp. low-calorie Italian dressing	10
Noncaloric sweetened tea or coffee	—
	290

Dinner

1 chicken breast, broiled	200
8 pods okra, boiled	30
1 cup squash, summer variety	40
1 slice whole wheat bread	60
½ cup applesauce, noncaloric sweetened	50
Noncaloric tea, sweetened	—
	380

Total calories for the day—1000

TUESDAY

Breakfast

Mix together:

½ cup strawberries, fresh or frozen	30
1 Tbsp. brewer's yeast	30
1 cup low-fat cottage cheese, topped with	205
2 tsp. vegetable-type bacon	90
Coffee, black	—
	355

Lunch

3 oz. calf liver, broiled	170
6 asparagus tips, canned	30
½ cup blackeyed peas	75
1 slice whole wheat bread	60
Noncaloric sweetened tea	—
	335

Dinner

3 oz. fresh shrimp, boiled	70
1 cup spinach, canned, topped with	55
1 egg, hard-cooked, sliced	75
Salad plate:	
½ tomato, sliced	15
3 young green onions	10
4 radishes, chopped	5
½ cup tapioca, cooked	80
Tea or decaffeinated coffee, black	—
	310

Total calories for the day—1000

Lord, I believe.

—Mark 9:24

WEDNESDAY

Breakfast

1 cup raw peaches, sliced, combined with	85
1 cup cooked farina and	100
½ cup skim milk	45
3 oz. dried beef	165
1 slice whole wheat bread, toasted	60
Coffee, black	—
	455

Lunch

1 chicken thigh, broiled	150
6 canned asparagus tips	30
½ cup eggplant, baked, topped with	10
2 Tbsp. wheat germ	30
½ cup fresh strawberries	30
Noncaloric tea, sweetened	—
	250

Dinner

3 oz. tuna, water-packed	130
*Fresh salad plate, topped with	60
2 Tbsp. low-fat cottage cheese	30
2 rye wafer crackers	45
2 pear halves, water-packed or non caloric sweetened	30
Noncaloric sweetened tea	—
	295

Total calories for the day—1000

THURSDAY

Breakfast

½ cantaloupe filled with	45
1 cup low-fat cottage cheese, topped with	205
2 tsp. vegetable-type bacon	90
Coffee, black	—
	340

Lunch

*1 cup cream of mushroom soup	85
3 oz. dry packed shrimp, boiled	100
½ cup carrots, cooked	20
1 med. tomato, sliced	30
1 slice whole wheat bread	60
Noncaloric sweetened tea	—
	295

Dinner

3 oz. roasted turkey	190
1 cup string beans	30
*Tomato aspic, 1 serving	40
1 slice whole wheat bread	60
4 oz. skim milk	45
	365

Total calories for the day—1000

Our fondest wish is to be weighed and found wanting.

FRIDAY

Breakfast

½ cup pineapple chunks, water-packed or noncaloric sweetened, topped with	50
½ cup low-fat cottage cheese	100
2 tsp. vegetable-type bacon	90
1 slice whole wheat bread, toasted	60
Coffee, black	—
	300

Lunch

3 oz. beef round steak, grilled	190
1 med. potato, baked	100
1 pat dietetic margarine	25
¼ med. head lettuce	20
½ raw tomato, sliced, with herb seasoning	15
1 (8 oz.) glass skim milk	85
	435

Dinner

Shrimp salad bowl:

1 egg. hard-cooked sliced	75
4 med. shrimp, broiled	90
½ cup lettuce, shredded	15
3 young green onions, chopped	10
Dash of sea salt	—
8 oz. glass chilled tomato juice, mixed with	60
1 ½ tsp. brewer's yeast	15
	265

Total calories for the day—1000

SATURDAY

Breakfast

1 cup vegetable juice mixed with	90
1½ tsp. brewer's yeast	15
½ cup low-fat cottage cheese	105
2 tsp. vegetable-type bacon	90
1 slice whole wheat bread, toasted	60
Coffee, black	—
	360

Lunch

3 oz. pink salmon, canned, broiled	120
½ cup tomatoes, chilled, canned	30
2 crackers, rye wafers	45
Relish dish:	
3 fresh green onions	10
4 small radishes	5
1 cup raw celery, chopped	20
1 cup raw carrots, sliced	50
*1 serving molded orange dessert	20
	300

Dinner

3 oz. turkey, roasted, dark & light meat	190
1 cup cauliflower, cooked	35
1 cup green beans	30
1 slice whole wheat bread, with	60
1 pat dietetic margarine	25
Noncaloric sweetened tea or decaffeinated coffee	—
	340

Total calories for the day—1000

SUNDAY

Breakfast

Mix together	
½ cup strawberries	30
1 med. banana, topped with	40
1 Tbsp. wheat germ	30
1 Tbsp. whipped nonfat dry milk solids	15
3 oz. lean ground beef patty, broiled	190
1 slice whole wheat bread, toasted	60
1 cup coffee, black	—
	365

Lunch

1 all beef frank, chopped, mixed with	110
1 cup sauerkraut, canned	45
1 apple, baked, noncaloric sweetened	80
1 slice whole wheat bread	60
Noncaloric sweetened tea	—
	295

Dinner

3 oz. beef sirloin, grilled	250
3 new potatoes, boiled	50
Dash of herb seasoning	—
1 cup spring salad	25
1 peach half, water-packed or noncaloric sweetened	15
	340

Total calories for the day—1000

Set a watch, O Lord, before my mouth.
—Psalm 141:3

MONDAY

Breakfast

½ cup salad fruit, water-packed or noncaloric sweetened, combined with	40
1 cup low-fat cottage cheese, topped with	205
2 tsp. vegetable-type bacon	90
Coffee, black	—
	335

Lunch

1 med. green pepper stuffed with	20
3 oz. lean ground beef, baked, served with	190
1 cup stewed tomatoes	55
1 slice whole wheat bread	60
½ cup fruit cocktail, water-packed or noncaloric sweetened	45
Noncaloric sweetened tea, hot or cold	—
	370

Dinner

3 oz. sole, broiled, lemon slice	140
1 med. potato, baked	100
1 pat. dietetic margarine	25
*1 cup green beans & celery julienne	30
1 glass noncaloric sweetened tea, iced	—
	295

Total calories for the day—1000

TUESDAY

Breakfast

8 oz. tomato juice, filled, mixed with	60
1½ tsp. brewer's yeast	15
1 egg, poached, topped with	75
2 tsp. vegetable-type bacon	90
1 slice whole wheat bread	60
Coffee, black	—
	300

Lunch

3 oz. fresh shrimp, boiled in herb seasoning	70
1 Tbsp. low-calorie catsup	20
1 cup English peas, cooked	110
*Fresh salad plate, 1 serving, topped with	55
*1 Tbsp. herb and oil dressing	15
Noncaloric sweetened tea, iced	—
	270

Dinner

½ lean chicken, charcoal-broiled	320
6 tips fresh asparagus, cooked	15
1 cup cauliflower, cooked	35
½ cup strawberries, fresh or frozen, topped with	30
2 Tbsp. low-fat cottage cheese	30
Noncaloric sweetened tea, hot	—
	430

Total calories for the day—1000

WEDNESDAY

Breakfast

½ cup salad fruits, water-packed or noncaloric sweetened	40
1 all-beef frankfurter	110
1 egg, scrambled with	75
1 Tbsp. wheat germ	15
1 slice whole wheat bread	60
1 Tbsp. dietetic jelly	—
1 cup coffee, black	—
	300

Lunch

4 oz. chicken, roasted	220
*Baked potato stuffed with low-fat cottage cheese	90
1 cup green beans	25
½ cup skim milk	45
	380

Dinner

5 oz. broiled trout, thin slice lemon	230
Salad: combine	
1 cup raw cabbage, grated	45
½ fresh raw green pepper, sliced	10
1 Tbsp. vinegar—dash of sea salt	5
½ cup strawberries	30
	320

Total calories for the day—1000

THURSDAY

Breakfast

½ med. grapefruit	110
2 buckwheat pancakes, 4" diam. topped with	90
2 tsp. vegetable-type bacon and	
1 Tbsp. dietetic jelly	90
1 glass (8 oz.) skim milk, mixed with	85
1½ tsp. brewer's yeast	15
Coffee, black	—
	390

Lunch

5 oz. trout, steamed, thin lemon slice	230
6 tips asparagus, fresh, boiled	15
½ tomato, sliced	15
3 fresh green onions	10
1 slice whole wheat bread	60
Noncaloric sweetened tea or coffee	—
	330

Dinner

3 oz. lean ground meat patty, broiled	190
½ cup green beans	15
*1 serving tomato aspic	40
2 Tbsp. low-fat yogurt, topped on	20
1 peach half, water-packed or noncaloric sweetened	15
Noncaloric sweetened tea, hot or cold	—
	280

Total calories for the day—1000

FRIDAY

Breakfast

1 cup Farina cooked, served with	100
4 oz. skim-milk	45
½ cup strawberries, topped with	30
2 Tbsp. low-fat cottage cheese	30
2 tsp. vegetable-type bacon	90
1 Tbsp. brewer's yeast	30
Coffee, black	—
	325

Lunch

1 med. fryer breast, broiled	200
6 asparagus tips	20
1 cup soft-shell squash, boiled	40
1 piece (2x2x¾") cornbread	80
1 glass noncaloric sweetened tea	—
	350

Dinner

*1 med. flounder Portuguese	180
1 cup eggplant, baked	25
½ cup raw cabbage, chopped, with herb seasoning	15
1 slice whole wheat bread	60
1 peach half, water-packed or noncaloric sweetened	15
2 Tbsp. low-fat cottage cheese	30
Noncaloric sweetened tea, hot or cold	—
	325

Total calories for the day—1000

SATURDAY

Breakfast

½ cup salad fruits, water-packed or noncaloric sweetened	40
1 cup bran flakes, enriched with	120
¼ cup wheat germ, topped with	70
1 cup skim milk	90
Noncaloric sweetened coffee, black	—
	320

Lunch

3 oz. lean ground beef, stuffed in	190
1 med. green pepper shell	20
Seasoned with celery salt	—
½ med. eggplant, baked	20
½ cup carrots, cooked	25
1 slice whole wheat bread	60
Noncaloric sweetened tea	—
	315

Dinner

3 oz. veal cutlet, broiled	175
1 med. potato, baked in jacket	100
1 cup green string beans	30
1 cup strawberries, fresh or frozen	60
Tea or decaffeinated coffee	—
	365

Total calories for the day—1000

SUNDAY

Breakfast

1 med. orange, sliced	80
3 oz. dried beef, mixed with	165
1 egg, scrambled	75
1 slice whole wheat bread, toasted	60
Coffee, black	—
	380

Lunch

*Mexican meatballs with soup, 1 serving	130
1 cup cabbage, boiled	50
½ cup squash, summer variety	20
*1 Stuffed baked apple	180
Noncaloric sweetened tea	—
	380

Dinner

3 oz. shrimp, boiled	100
½ cup broccoli, boiled, topped with	25
1 Tbsp. toasted wheat germ	15
1 med. raw tomato, sliced	35
2 young green onions	5
1 slice whole wheat bread	60
Tea or decaffeinated coffee	—
	240

Total calories for the day—1000

MONDAY

Breakfast

½ cantaloupe, filled with	45
1 cup low-fat cottage cheese, topped with	205
2 tsp. vegetable-bacon	90
Coffee, black	—
	340

Lunch

*1 cup cream of mushroom soup	85
3 oz. dry-packed shrimp, boiled	100
½ cup carrots, cooked	20
1 med. tomato, sliced	30
1 slice whole wheat bread	60
Noncaloric sweetened tea	—
	295

Dinner

3 oz. roasted turkey	190
1 cup string beans	30
*Tomato aspic, 1 serving	40
1 slice whole wheat bread	60
4 oz. skim milk	45
	365

Total calories for the day—1000

The easiest place to stay on a diet plan is in front of a mirror.

TUESDAY

Breakfast

½ cup salad fruits, water-packed or noncaloric sweetened	40
1 cup bran flakes, enriched with	120
¼ cup wheat germ, topped with	70
1 cup skim milk	90
Noncaloric sweetened to taste	—
Coffee, black	—
	320

Lunch

3 oz. lean ground beef, stuffed in	190
1 med. green pepper shell	20
Seasoned with celery salt	—
½ med. eggplant, baked	20
½ cup carrots, cooked	25
1 slice whole wheat bread	60
Noncaloric sweetened tea	—
	315

Dinner

3 oz. veal cutlet, broiled	175
1 med. potato, baked in jacket	100
1 cup green string beans	30
1 cup strawberries, fresh or frozen	60
Tea or decaffeinated coffee	
	365

Total calories for the day—1000

WEDNESDAY

Breakfast

½ grapefruit, broiled and topped with	110
1 tsp. low-calorie cranberry sauce	5
3 oz. dried beef	165
1 slice whole wheat bread, toasted	60
1 cup coffee, black	—
	340

Lunch

*Vegetable-stuffed beef roll-up, 1 serving	325
½ cup green beans	15
½ med. raw tomato, sliced	15
1 glass noncaloric sweetened tea, iced	—
	355

Dinner

3 oz. chicken livers, broiled	115
1 cup cabbage, boiled, topped with	50
2 tsp. vegetable-type bacon	90
1 cup eggplant, baked	25
½ cup cling peaches, water-packed or noncaloric sweetened	40
1 glass noncaloric sweetened tea, iced	—
	305

Total calories for the day—1000

A man hopes that there are no more lean years for him, but a woman hopes that hers are ahead.

THURSDAY

Breakfast

Combine:	
1 cup raw peaches, sliced	85
1 cup cooked Farina	100
½ cup skim milk	45
3 oz. dried beef	165
1 slice whole wheat bread, toasted	60
Coffee, black	—
	455

Lunch

1 chicken thigh, broiled	150
6 canned asparagus tips	30
½ cup eggplant, baked, topped with	10
2 Tbsp. wheat germ	30
½ cup fresh strawberries	30
Noncaloric sweetened tea	—
	250

Dinner

3 oz. tuna, water-packed	130
*Fresh salad plate, topped with	60
2 Tbsp. low-fat cottage cheese	30
2 rye wafer crackers	45
2 pear halves, water-packed, or noncaloric sweetened	30
Noncaloric sweetened tea	—
	295

Total calories for the day—1000

FRIDAY

Breakfast
Combine:

½ cup salad fruit, water-packed or noncaloric sweetened	40
1 cup low-fat cottage cheese, topped with	205
2 tsp. vegetable-type bacon	90
Coffee, black	—
	335

Lunch

1 med. green pepper, stuffed with	20
3 oz. lean ground beef, baked with	190
1 cup stewed tomatoes	55
1 slice whole wheat bread	60
½ cup fruit cocktail, water-packed or noncaloric sweetened	45
Noncaloric sweetened tea, hot or cold	—
	370

Dinner

3 oz. sole, broiled, topped	140
¼ of med. lemon, sliced	
1 med. potato, baked	100
1 pat dietetic margarine	25
*1 cup green beans & celery julienne	30
1 glass noncaloric sweetened tea	—
	295

Total calories for the day—1000

You may find yourself way out in front if you exceed the feed limit.

SATURDAY

Breakfast
½ grapefruit	110
1 egg, scrambled with	75
1 all-beef frank, chopped, and	110
1 Tbsp. wheat germ	15
1 slice whole wheat bread, toasted	60
1 cup coffee, black	—
	370

Lunch
1 cup canned bouillon	30
3 oz. veal cutlet, broiled	175
*Fruit delight mold, 1 serving, served on	90
¼ head lettuce, shredded	20
Noncaloric sweetened tea	—
	315

Dinner
3 oz. shrimp, fresh-boiled, served with	70
*1 Tbsp. low-calorie seafood cocktail sauce	5
1 med. potato, baked	105
1 pat dietetic margarine	25
*Sunshine salad, 1 serving	20
1 slice whole wheat bread	60
½ cup fruit cocktail, water-packed	30
Noncaloric sweetened tea	—
	315

Total calories for the day—1000

Eat so much as is sufficient for thee.
—*Proverbs 25:16*

SUNDAY

Breakfast

½ cup salad fruits, water-packed or noncaloric sweetened	40
1 all-beef frankfurter	110
1 egg, scrambled with	75
1 Tbsp. wheat germ	15
1 slice whole wheat bread	60
1 Tbsp. dietetic jelly	—
1 cup coffee, black	—
	300

Lunch

4 oz. chicken, roasted	220
*Baked potato stuffed with cottage cheese	90
1 cup green beans	25
½ cup skim milk	45
	380

Dinner

5 oz. broiled trout, sliced lemon	230
Salad: combine	
1 cup raw cabbage, grated	45
½ raw green pepper, sliced	10
1 Tbsp. vinegar—dash of sea salt	5
½ cup strawberries	30
Noncaloric sweetened tea	—

Total calories for the day—1000

Ask, and it shall be given you.

—Matthew 7:7

MONDAY

Breakfast

1 cup vegetable juice, mixed with	90
1½ tsp. brewer's yeast	15
½ cup low-fat cottage cheese	105
2 tsp. vegetable-type bacon	90
1 slice whole wheat bread, toasted	60
Coffee, black	—
	360

Lunch

3 oz. pink salmon, canned, broiled	120
½ cup tomatoes, chilled, canned	30
2 crackers, rye wafers	45
Relish dish	
3 fresh green onions	10
4 radishes, small	5
1 cup raw celery, chopped	20
1 cup raw carrots, sliced	50
*1 serving molded orange dessert	20
Noncaloric sweetened tea, hot or cold	—
	300

Dinner

3 oz. turkey, roasted, dark & white meat	190
1 cup cauliflower, cooked	35
1 cup green beans	30
1 slice whole wheat bread, topped with	60
1 pat dietetic margarine	25
Noncaloric sweetened tea or decaffeinated coffee	—
	340

Total calories for the day—1000

TUESDAY

Breakfast

½ cup purple plums, water-packed or noncaloric sweetened	50
1 slice whole wheat bread, toasted, topped with	60
1 pat dietetic margarine, and	25
2 tsp. vegetable-type bacon	90
1 cup skim milk	85
Coffee, black	—
	310

Lunch

1 cup noodles, cooked, topped with	100
3 oz. fresh shrimp, boiled	70
4 oz. fresh lettuce, chopped	20
1 med. raw tomato, sliced	35
½ cup tapioca, cooked	80
Tea of coffee	—

Dinner

3 oz. sirloin beef, broiled	250
½ cup peas and carrots, canned	35
1 cup raw cabbage, chopped, seasoned with lemon juice	25 —
2 ginger snaps	40
½ cup fruit cocktail, water-packed or noncaloric sweetened	35
Noncaloric sweetened tea or coffee	—
	385

Total calories for the day—1000

WEDNESDAY

Breakfast

2½ sliced pineapple, water-packed or noncaloric sweetened, topped with	65
1 cup low-fat cottage cheese	205
1 slice whole wheat bread, toasted	60
Coffee, black	—
	330

Lunch

8 oz. flounder, steamed	220
Salad:	
4 oz. fresh lettuce, chopped	20
½ med. raw tomato, sliced	20
2 fresh green onions	10
½ pickle	10
2 tsp. low-calorie Italian dressing	10
Noncaloric sweetened tea or coffee	—
	290

Dinner

1 chicken breast, broiled	200
8 pods okra, boiled	30
1 cup squash, summer variety	40
1 slice whole wheat bread	60
½ cup applesauce, noncaloric sweetened	50
Noncaloric sweetened tea	—
	380

Total calories for the day—1000

THURSDAY

Breakfast

½ med. grapefruit	110
2 buckwheat pancakes, 4" diam., topped with	90
2 tsp. vegetable-type bacon, and	90
1 Tbsp. dietetic jelly	—
1 glass (8 oz.) skim milk, mixed with	85
1½ tsp. brewer's yeast	15
Coffee, black	—
	390

Lunch

5 oz. trout, steamed, lemon slice	230
6 fresh asparagus tips, boiled	15
½ tomato, sliced	15
3 fresh green onions	10
1 slice whole wheat bread	60
Noncaloric sweetened tea or coffee	—
	330

Dinner

3 oz. lean ground meat patty, broiled	190
½ cup green beans	15
*1 serving Tomato aspic	40
2 Tbsp. low-fat yogurt, topped on	20
1 peach half, water-packed or noncaloric sweetened	15
Noncaloric sweetened tea, hot or cold	—
	280

Total calories for the day—1000

FRIDAY

Breakfast

8 oz. tomato juice, chilled, mixed with	60
1½ tsp. brewer's yeast	15
1 egg, poached, topped with	75
2 tsp. vegetable-type bacon	90
1 slice whole wheat bread	60
Coffee, black	—
	300

Lunch

3 oz. fresh shrimp, boiled in herb seasoning	70
1 Tbsp. low-calorie catsup	20
1 cup English peas, cooked	110
*Fresh salad plate, 1 serving, topped with	55
*1 Tbsp. herb and oil dressing	15
Noncaloric sweetened tea, iced	—
	270

Dinner

½ lean chicken, charcoal-broiled	320
6 fresh-cooked asparagus tips	15
1 cup cauliflower, cooked	35
½ cup strawberries, fresh or frozen, topped with	30
2 Tbsp. low-fat cottage cheese	30
Noncaloric sweetened tea, hot	—
	430

Total calories for the day—1000

SATURDAY

Breakfast

1 cup blackberries, mixed with	85
1 cup low-fat cottage cheese	205
1 slice whole wheat bread, toasted	60
Coffee, black	—
	350

Lunch

4 oz. lean ground beef, broiled with	235
½ cup carrots	25
Dash celery salt	—
½ cup tomatoes, plus ½ cup water	30
Saltine crackers, 4-2½"	60
Noncaloric sweetened tea	—
	350

Dinner

1 med. fresh perch, pan-fried, in Teflon pan	110
1 med. potato, baked in jacket	100
*1 cup spring salad	45
1 peach half, water-packed or noncaloric sweetened, topped with	15
2 Tbsp. low-fat cottage cheese	30
Coffee or tea	—
	300

Total calories for the day—1000

The weight of a man's years invariably settles around his beltline.

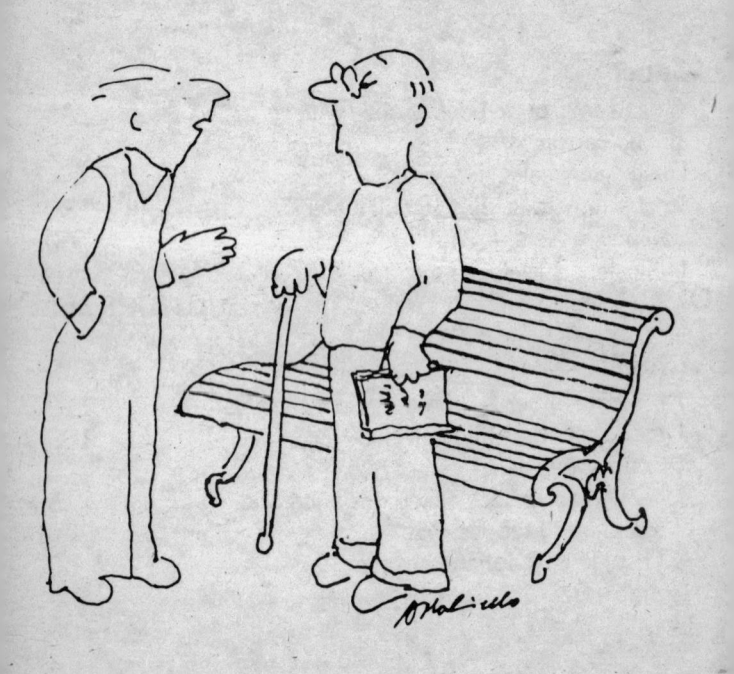

"My wife says she's pushing 115 pounds. I guess she pulls the other 30."

4

UNTHOUGHT-OF-RECIPES

Get the right balance
of protein, fat, and carbohydrates
in your low-calorie diet

- Suggested recipes
- Using your own recipes
- Low-calorie recipes for 1000-calorie and 500-calorie diets

500-CALORIE RECIPE INDEX

Tomato Sauce
Stuffed Celery
Mock Spaghetti w/Meatballs
Stuffed Pepper
Chipped Beef Roll
Liver/Beefburger
Chow Mein Special
Turkey Salad
Tomato Aspic
Raw Vegetable Mold
Yogurt Dressing
Cauliflower in Sauce
Applesauce Gelatin
Carrot and Cottage Cheese Salad
Tomato Baked Fish
Consomme Bouquetiere
Cold Shrimp Bisque
Chili Marvel
Swiss Steak
Dried Beef Rolls or Turkey Roll
Clear Onion Soup

USE YOUR OWN FAVORITE RECIPES!

Low-calorie recipes of your own choosing can be adapted to your 500- or 1000-calorie plan by carefully following these steps:

1. Use only foods on the allowable list.
2. Look up the calorie listing for each item in the recipe.
3. Add up the caloric values of all items, then divide the total for the recipe by the number of servings.
4. Fit your recipe into the daily plan, always taking care not to exceed the total allowable calories.

EXAMPLE:
Low-Calorie Whipped Cream

¼ cup evaporated milk	90
(chilled in freezer for a few hours)	
¾ tsp. unflavored gelatin	15
½ cup boiling water	—
1½ tsp. noncaloric sweetener	—
1½ tsp. lemon juice	trace
1½ tsp. vanilla	trace
Total calories for the recipe—1 cup:	105
Total calories per 1 serving—4 Tbsp.:	25

1. Place evaporated milk into refrigerator tray and chill until ice crystals begin to form around edges; also chill a mixing bowl and rotary beaters.
2. Soak gelatin in cold water for about 5 minutes. Pour boiling water over and stir until gelatin is dissolved.
3. Spoon chilled evaporated milk from tray into chilled mixing bowl.
4. Add noncaloric sweetener and flavoring. Beat rapidly for about 10 minutes, until thick and creamy.
5. Add gelatin mixture and lemon juice, and continue beating until of whipped-cream consistency.
6. Refrigerate in the freezer compartment for at least one hour. Beat again immediately before serving.

TOMATO SAUCE

Yield: 1½ cups

1 cup tomatoes
1 bouillon cube
1 onion, minced
1 Tbsp. lemon juice
1 Tbsp. Worcestershire sauce
1 bay leaf
Noncaloric liquid sweetener, to taste
Salt, sea or vegetable, and pepper to taste

1. Dissolve bouillion cube in ¼ cup boiling water.
2. Add other ingredients and simmer 5 minutes.
3. Season and sweeten to taste.
   Total caloric value: 2 Tbsp.—5 calories

STUFFED CELERY

Yield: 12 pieces

2 large stalks celery, 12 inches long
3 Tbsp. low-fat cottage cheese
1 vegetable broth tablet
1 oz. Roquefort cheese
1 tsp. chives, chopped
Few drops Worcestershire sauce

1. Cut celery into 2-inch lengths. Place in icewater while preparing the cheese mixture.
2. Dissolve the broth tablet in 2 Tbsp. boiling water. Add the Roquefort cheese and Worcestershire sauce. Stir well.
3. Sprinkle chives into the cottage cheese. Combine with the Roquefort mixture.
4. Dry celery and stuff with the cheese mixture. Total caloric value: one 2-inch slice—15 calories.

MOCK SPAGHETTI WITH MEATBALLS

Yield: 1 serving

1 cup bean sprouts, heated and well-drained
4 Tbsp. mock spaghetti sauce
Simmer until hot and serve with
3½ oz. ground round steak, roll into three meatballs and broil in oven.

1. Cover broiled meatballs with bean sprouts.
2. Top with mock spaghetti sauce and serve.
   Total caloric value in 1 serving: 290 calories

MOCK SPAGHETTI SAUCE

Yield: 1½ cups

1 cup vinegar
½ cup catsup
1 clove of garlic
2 Tbsp. Worcestershire sauce
1 tsp. liquid noncaloric sweetener
1 tsp. dry mustard
½ tsp. Tabasco sauce
1 tsp. salt, sea or vegetable

Mix together all ingredients and simmer 10 minutes in a saucepan.
   Total caloric value: 1 Tbsp.—10 calories

STUFFED PEPPER

Yield: 1 serving

1 med. green pepper, parboiled
3 oz. lean ground beef
1 fresh green onion, chopped

1. Mix onion and ground round beef in parboiled green pepper shell.
2. Place in a covered baking dish in a 350-degree oven and cook until done, about 20 minutes.

Total caloric value: 1 serving—215 calories

CHIPPED BEEF ROLLS

Yield: 12 beef rolls

¼ cup low-fat cottage cheese
2 Tbsps. onions, grated
¼ tsp. Worcestershire sauce
1/8 tsp. pepper
½ tsp. brewer's yeast
12 slices chipped beef, 3 oz.

1. Mix together the cottage cheese, onion, Worcestershire sauce, pepper, and brewer's yeast.
2. Place a tsp. of the mixture on each slice of beef. Roll tightly and fasten with cocktail picks.
3. Chill before serving.

Total caloric value: 1 beef roll—20 calories

May you live all the days of your life.

—Swift

BAKED TOMATO WITH MEAT STUFFING

Yield: 4 servings

4 med. tomatoes
½ lb. ground round
¼ cup melba toast crumbs
¼ cup wheat germ
2 Tbsp. cold water
2 Tbsp. onion, chopped
1/8 tsp. basil
¼ tsp. Worcestershire sauce
¼ tsp. salt

1. Remove tops from tomato and scoop out the pulp. Salt and pepper the inside of the tomato.
2. Add ground meat and onions in heavy skillet together—stir with fork until meat and onions brown.
3. Remove meat from heat, stir in the toast crumbs, wheat germ, and remaining ingredients. Mix well.
4. Fill tomatoes with meat mixture, place in shallow baking dish, and add ¼ cup hot water.
5. Bake in 375 degrees oven for 25 minutes.

Total caloric value: 1 serving—225 calories

Health is the vital principle of bliss.

—Thomson

LIVER/BEEF BURGER

Yield: 2 servings

3 oz. lean ground beef
3 oz. beef liver, chopped
3 Tbsp. raw onions, chopped
1 Tbsp. raw parsley, chopped

1. Mix all ingredients together and shape into two patties.
2. Broil on each side until golden brown.

Total caloric value: 1 serving—185 calories

CHOW MEIN SPECIAL

Yield: 2 servings

3 oz. veal cutlet, cut in small cube
1 clove of garlic
1 can (2 cups) soy sprouts, drain, save liquid
6 young green onions, chopped
2 large celery stalks, sliced

1. Rub garlic into skillet with nonstick finish, discard remainder of clove.
2. Brown cubed veal, cook slowly for 5 minutes; drain off fat.
3. Add chopped onions and ½ cup bean sprout liquid, cook 1 minute.
4. Add sliced celery stalks, cover pan; cook 10 minutes over very low heat.
5. Add bean sprouts, stir, and cook 5 more minutes, covered.

Total caloric value: 1 serving—170 calories

TURKEY SALAD

Yield: 3 servings

6 oz. turkey, roasted; diced
1 cup celery, diced
½ med. lemon, juiced
3 Tbsp. yogurt dressing
½ tsp. ground black pepper
Salt to taste

Gently combine all ingredients, serve on romaine lettuce leaf.
  Total caloric value: 1 serving—150 calories

TOMATO ASPIC

1 Tbsp. unflavored gelatin
2 onion slices
2 cups tomato juice
1 Tbsp. vinegar
¼ tsp. salt, sea or vegetable
½ bay leaf
Few drops of Tabasco sauce
Lettuce leaves

1. Add the onion, salt, Tabasco, and bay leaf to tomato juice. Simmer for 10 minutes.
2. Soften gelatin in ¼ cup cold water and dissolve in hot tomato juice mixture.
3. Add vinegar, then strain.
4. Pour into mold and chill until firm. Serve on lettuce.
  Total caloric value: 1 serving—40 calories

RAW VEGETABLE MOLD

1 envelope unflavored gelatin
1 bouillon cube
1 Tbsp. lemon juice
¼ tsp. salt, sea or vegetable
¾ cup cabbage, chopped
¾ cup raw carrots, shredded
½ cup celery, chopped
Salad greens

1. Soften the gelatin in ½ cup cold water, then dissolve over low heat or hot water.
2. Dissolve the bouillon cube in 1 cup boiling water.
3. Combine the gelatin and bouillon. Add lemon juice and salt.
4. Chill to the consistency of unbeaten egg whites. Fold in the vegetables. Pour into salad mold and chill until firm. Serve on salad greens.

Total caloric value: 1 serving—25 calories

YOGURT DRESSING

Yield: 1 cup

1 cup plain low-fat yogurt
3 tsp. lemon juice
1 tsp salt
¼ tsp. prepared mustard

1. Mix lemon juice and salt, blending in mustard.
2. Gradually add to the yogurt, blending thoroughly.
3. Chill for at least ½ hour before using.

Total caloric value: 1 Tbsp.—10 calories.

CAULIFLOWER SAUCE

Boil and drain 1 cup cauliflower. Place in casserole. Pour over cauliflower the following sauce and brown in oven.

Sauce:
1 Tbsp. flour
½ cup nonfat dry milk solids
1/8 tsp. white pepper
½ tsp. salt
1 cup water

1. In a saucepan, mix the flour, dry milk, salt, and pepper.
2. Add the water and beat until smooth.
3. Cook over low heat, stirring constantly until the sauce thickens.

Total caloric value: 1 cup cauliflower with 2 Tbsp. sauce—55 calories.

APPLESAUCE GELATIN

Yield: 4 servings

1 envelope unflavored gelatin
3 small apples
½ tsp. vanilla extract
1 Tbsp. lemon juice
1 tsp. liquid noncaloric sweetener
4 sprigs mint

1. Cook apples in 1 cup water until tender. Rub through a sieve or mash. Add vanilla.
2. Soften gelatin in ¼ cup of cold water. Dissolve in ¾ cup boiling water. Add noncaloric sweetener and lemon juice.
3. Combine gelatin and applesauce. Heap in serving glasses and chill until firm.

Total caloric value: 1 serving—70 calories

CARROT AND COTTAGE CHEESE SALAD

Yield: 1 serving

½ cup carrots, grated
1 Tbsp. cottage cheese
*1 Tbsp. yogurt dressing
Chopped onion to taste
Chopped caraway seeds to taste
Lettuce leaves

1. Blend the cottage cheese with the onion and caraway seeds.
2. Lightly toss the carrots with this mixture.
3. Arrange on lettuce leaf and sprinkle yogurt dressing over the salad.

Total caloric value: 1 serving—40 calories

TOMATO BAKED FISH

Yield: 6 servings

2 pounds haddock
3 tsp. salt, sea or vegetable
½ tsp. pepper
1 tsp. vegetable salad oil
¼ cup onion, chopped
¼ cup celery, chopped
1 med. green pepper, chopped
2 cups tomatoes, canned
¼ tsp. garlic powder
1 tsp. chili powder
1 Tbsp. Worcestershire sauce
1 bay leaf

1. Place the fish in a baking dish and sprinkle with 2 tsp. of the salt and ¼ tsp. of the pepper. Refrigerate while preparing the sauce.

2. Heat the oil in a heavy saucepan; saute the onion, celery, and green pepper until lightly browned. Add the remaining salt and pepper.
3. Stir in the tomatoes, garlic powder, Worcestershire sauce, and bay leaf. Cook over low heat 20 minutes, stirring frequently.
4. Remove bay leaf from the sauce and puree the mixture in an electric blender or force through a sieve.
5. Pour the sauce over the fish. Bake in a 350-degree oven for 50 minutes or until the fish is flaky. Baste frequently.

Total caloric value: 1 serving—135 calories

CHILI MARVEL

Yield: 3 servings

4 medium tomatoes, chopped, blend in a blender
1 med. raw onion, chopped
6 oz. ground round steak
1 bouillon cube
¼ cup hot water.
Salt, pepper and chili powder to taste

1. Brown meat and onions in a heavy kettle, stirring with a fork. It will not be necessary to grease pan.
2. Dissolve bouillon cube in hot water.
3. When meat and onions are browned, pour off excess fat, add bouillon, and tomatoes.
4. Add seasoning to taste and simmer until done, about 30 minutes.

Total caloric value: 1 serving—155 calories.

102
SWISS STEAK

Yield: 1 serving

3 oz. veal cutlet
Garlic bud
3 young green onions, chopped
½ med. tomato, chopped
¼ cup raw carrots, chopped
½ cup consomme
Season to taste

1. Remove all excess fat from cutlet.
2. Place veal cutlet on broiler, and quickly brown each side.
3. Place chopped onions, carrot, and tomato in blender. Blend until pureed.
4. Rub bottom and sides of casserole with garlic clove.
5. Place cutlet in casserole. Top with pureed mixture and consomme. Season to taste.
6. Cover casserole and bake in a slow oven (275 degrees) until meat is tender, about one hour.

Total caloric value: 1 serving—225 calories

DRIED BEEF ROLLS OR TURKEY ROLL

Yield: 3 servings

6 thin slices dried beef, 1½ oz.
6 Tbsp. low-fat cottage cheese
Dash of Worcestershire sauce

1. Season the cottage cheese with Worcestershire sauce.
2. Roll the beef slices into cornucopias and fill with the cheese.

Total caloric value: 1 serving—35 calories

VARIANT

1. Substitute 6 thin slices of turkey for the dried beef.
   Total caloric value: 1 serving—30 calories

CLEAR ONION SOUP

Yield: 2 servings

2 vegetable bouillon tablets
2 cups boiling water
1 med. onion, thinly sliced

1. Dissolve the bouillon tablets in the boiling water.
2. Add the sliced onions and simmer over low heat until onions are tender.
   Total caloric value: 1 cup—15 calories

CONSOMME BOUQUETIERE

Yield: 4 servings

1 medium carrot
6 string beans
¼ cup green peas
4 chicken bouillon cubes

1. Slice carrot into thin round circles.
2. Cut beans into ½ inch lengths.
3. Mix together the carrot, beans, and peas. Cover with 5 cups of boiling water and boil, uncovered, until tender.
4. Add the bouillon cubes and stir until dissolved. Serve immediately.
   Total caloric value: 1 serving—25 calories

COLD SHRIMP BISQUE

Yield: 4 servings

½ pound shrimp, cooked and chopped
½ medium cucumber, diced
4 cups buttermilk
1 Tbsp. dill pickle, chopped
1 Tbsp. prepared mustard
1 Tbsp. nonfat dry milk solids
1/8 tsp. liquid noncaloric sweetener
1 tsp. salt, sea or vegetable
½ tsp. brewer's yeast

Mix together all ingredients. Chill before serving.
  Total caloric value: 1 serving—140 calories

More people commit suicide with a fork than with any other weapon.

SERENITY PRAYER

God grant me the serenity to accept the things I cannot change,
The courage to change the things I can,
And the wisdom to know the difference.

1000-CALORIE RECIPE INDEX

Tomato Aspic
Flounder Portugese
Molded Orange Dessert
Fresh Salad Plate
Spring Salad
Herb & Oil Dressing
Cream of Mushroom Soup
Baked Potato Stuffed with Cottage Cheese
Green Beans and Celery Julienne
Fruit Delight Mold
Stuffed Baked Apple
Mexican Meatballs with Soup
Vegetable-Stuffed Beef Roll-Up
Sunshine Salad
Low-Calorie Seafood Cocktail Sauce

For I the Lord thy God will hold thy right hand, saying unto thee, Fear not: I will help thee.

—Isaiah 41:13

TOMATO ASPIC

Yield: 4 servings

1 Tbsp. unflavored gelatin
2 onion slices
2 cups tomato juice
1 Tbsp. vinegar
¼ tsp. salt, sea or vegetable
½ bay leaf
Few drops Tabasco sauce
4 lettuce leaves

1. Add the onion, salt, Tabasco, and bay leaf to tomato juice.
2. Soften gelatin in ¼ cup cold water and dissolve in hot tomato juice mixture.
3. Add vinegar, then strain.
4. Pour into mold and chill until firm.

Serve on lettuce leaf.
  Total caloric value: 1 serving—40 calories

FLOUNDER PORTUGUESE

Yield: 1 serving
Flounder—small, about ¼ lb.
½ cup onions, diced
1 cup tomato juice
1 tsp. vinegar
1 Tbsp. parsley, chopped
1 Tbsp. lemon juice

1. Place fish in baking dish.
2. Cover with onions, tomato juice, vinegar, and parsley.
3. Bake in hot (450°) oven for 15 minutes.
4. Sprinkle with lemon juice and serve.

  Total caloric value: 1 serving—180 calories

MOLDED ORANGE DESSERT

Yield: 2 servings

1 envelope unflavored gelatin
2 Tbsp. orange juice
1 cup boiling water
Rind of ½ orange, grated
½ tsp. liquid noncaloric sweetener

1. Soften the gelatin in the orange juice. Dissolve in the boiling water.
2. Add the noncaloric sweetener and the grated orange rind. Pour into individual molds and chill until firm.

Total caloric value: 1 serving—20 calories

FRESH SALAD PLATE

Yield: 1 serving

4 oz. lettuce—fresh, shredded
½ med. tomato—raw, sliced
2 fresh green onions
½ large dill pickle

1. Clean and prepare vegetables
2. Arrange on salad plate.

Total caloric value: 1 serving—55 calories

SPRING SALAD

Yield: 3 servings

Gently toss together:
¼ head lettuce, shredded
½ ripe tomato, cubed
½ cup raw cauliflower, chopped
½ cup celery, diced
½ cup string beans well-drained and chilled
Season with sea salt
   Total caloric value: 1 serving—25 calories

HERB & OIL DRESSING

Yield: 2 cups

Mix together the following:
½ cup soybean oil (corn, cottonseed, safflower, or sunflower seed oil may be used).
¼ cup apple cider vinegar
1 cup water
1 garlic bud, minced
1 tsp. herb seasoning
   Total caloric value: 1 Tbsp.—15 calories

CREAM OF MUSHROOM SOUP

Yield: 6 servings

1 pat dietetic margarine
1 med. onion
2 cups mushrooms, chopped
4 cups chicken consomme
¼ tsp. pepper
1 cup skim milk
1 Tbsp. parsley, chopped

1. Melt the butter in a saucepan.
2. Saute the onion and mushrooms until lightly browned and add the consomme and pepper.
3. Add milk, then cover and cook over low heat 30 minutes.
4. Garnish with parsley.

Total caloric value: 1 serving—85 calories

BAKED POTATO STUFFED WITH COTTAGE CHEESE

Yield: 6 servings

3 med. potatoes, baked
½ cup skim milk
1 cup low-fat cottage cheese
Salt, pepper, paprika

1. Cut baked potatoes in half, lengthwise, scoop out the potato.
2. Mash and heat in the milk, cottage cheese, and seasoning.
3. Fill the potato shell with the cottage cheese mixture and sprinkle with paprika.
4. Place on baking sheet and bake at 400° until the top is brown.

Total caloric value: 1 serving—90 calories

GREEN BEANS & CELERY JULIENNE

2 cups green beans, thinly sliced
1 cup julienne of celery of the same size
1 Tbsp. dietetic margarine

1. Cook beans and celery for a short time separately (vegetables should be a little crisp).
2. Combine the vegetables and margarine; serve.

Total caloric value: 1 serving—30 calories

110
FRUIT DELIGHT MOLD

Yield: 8 servings

1 can water-packed fruit (peaches, pears)
2 Tbsp. unflavored gelatin
To taste—noncaloric lemon extract
1 cup skim milk
2 cups low-fat cottage cheese
2 Tbsp. chives, diced
½ cup celery, diced
¼ cup radishes, diced
¼ cup carrots, diced

1. Drain water packed fruit, add water to liquid to make 2 cups.
2. Heat to boiling and dissolve 1 Tbsp. of gelatin, add noncaloric extract, and chill until syrupy.
3. Arrange fruit attractively in bottom of a 1½-quart mold. Spoon gelatin over fruit and chill until firm.
4. Combine remaining unflavored gelatin and milk. Stir over low heat until gelatin dissolves.
5. Beat in cottage cheese, chives, celery, radishes, and carrots. Spoon mixture over fruit in mold. Chill until firm.
6. Unmold and garnish.

Total caloric value: 1 serving—90 calories

STUFFED BAKED APPLE

Yield: 2 servings

2 baking apples, washed and cored
1/8 tsp. cinnamon
2 tsp. liquid noncaloric sweetener
1 cup low-fat cottage cheese

1. Peel skin down from the top. Leave a portion around the base of the apple.
2. Place each apple in a shallow custard cup.
3. Stir noncaloric sweetener and cinnamon into ¼ cup water; pour over the apples.
4. Bake at 375° F. about 45 minutes or until apples are tender.
5. Serve hot with ½ cup cottage cheese topping.

Total caloric value: 1 serving—180 calories

MEXICAN MEATBALLS WITH SOUP

Yield: 6 servings

Meatballs:
¾ lb. ground round beef
1 egg, well-beaten
¼ cup onion, chopped
1 Tbsp. parsley, chopped
¼ tsp. mint, chopped
¼ tsp. marjoram
¼ tsp. salt, sea or vegetable
1/8 tsp. pepper
½ tsp. brewer's yeast
1½ tsp. unbleached white
  flour for dusting

Soup:
- 2 beef bouillon cubes
- 1 egg, well-beaten
- 1 tsp. salt, sea or vegetable
- ½ tsp. brewer's yeast
- 1 small bay leaf, crushed
- 1 cup canned tomatoes

1. Mix together all meat ingredients. Shape into 1-inch balls and dust with unbleached flour.
2. Dissolve bouillon cubes in 4 cups of boiling water. Drop meatballs into the water.
3. Cover and simmer for 30 minutes.
4. Stir in the salt, crushed bay leaf, and tomatoes. Cover and cook an additional 45 minutes.
5. Just before serving, stir in the well-beaten egg and brewer's yeast.

Total caloric value: 1 serving—130 calories

VEGETABLE-STUFFED BEEF ROLL-UP

Yield: 6 servings

- 6 - 3 oz. beef flank steaks
- 1 tsp. sea salt
- ¼ tsp. pepper
- ¼ cup low-calorie French dressing
- 1½ cup raw carrots, shredded
- ¼ cup chopped onion
- 1 med. raw green pepper, chopped
- 1 cup raw diced celery
- ¼ cup water

1. Sprinkle meat with the sea salt and pepper.
2. Marinate in low-calorie French dressing 30 to 60 minutes at room temperature.

3. In saucepan, simmer vegetables in small amount of water about 10 minutes. Drain.
4. Drain steaks; place about ⅓ cup vegetable mixture on each steak. Roll up and secure with wooden picks.
5. Grill steaks for 20-25 minutes, turning occasionally, until the desired doneness.

Total Caloric value: 1 serving—325 calories

SUNSHINE SALAD

Yield: 4 servings

½ cup carrots, shredded
½ cup celery, chopped
¼ cup bell pepper, chopped
1 bouillon cube
1 cup hot water
1 pkg. Knox gelatin
½ cup cold water
1/8 tsp. sea salt

1. Soften gelatin in cold water.
2. In a large bowl, melt bouillon cube in hot water.
3. Mix together, add salt, stir until gelatin is dissolved.
4. Cool, add vegetables when mixture begins to congeal.
5. Pour into mold and chill.

Serve on crisp lettuce leaves.

Total caloric value: 1 serving—20 calories

Some people have developed bay windows from eating too much see-food.

114
LOW-CALORIE SEAFOOD COCKTAIL SAUCE

Yield: 1½ cups

2 Tbsp. malt vinegar
¼ tsp. Worcestershire sauce
¼ tsp. Tabasco sauce
Pinch of sea salt
3 Tbsp. low-calorie catsup
2 Tbsp. horseradish
3 Tbsp. chili sauce

1. Add the salt to the vinegar, and stir in the Worcestershire sauce.
2. Mix in the Tabasco, horseradish, chili sauce, and catsup. Blend.

Total caloric value: 1 Tbsp.—5 calories

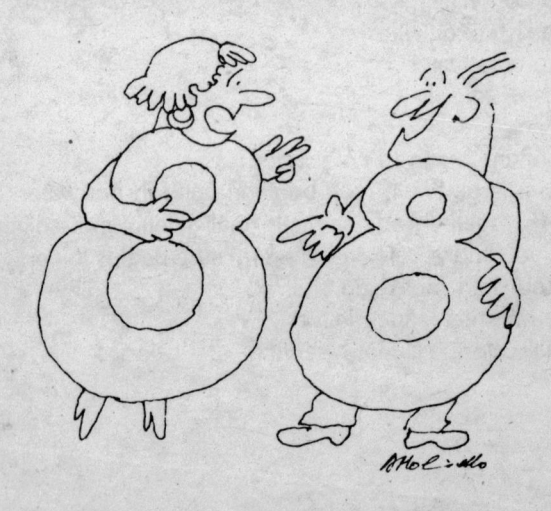

Some people are no good at counting calories, and they have the figures to prove it.

5

SLENDERIZING SNACKS

51 ways to feel like you're cheating— on 200 calories or less!

- Snacking in your diet
- 200-calorie snacks
- 100-calorie snacks

SLIMMING SNACK SUGGESTIONS

Many persons following a strict weight-correction diet plan or carefully planning their meals to control metabolic problems such as hypoglycemia (low blood sugar) or diabetes (high blood sugar) welcome a snack at bedtime or between meals.

This section contains 51 snack suggestions which will provide you with a high-protein boost at bedtime or between meals. Other meals during the day can be adjusted downward in calories to make room for the extra calories in your snack— approximately 100 calories or approximately 200 calories. If this system fits your needs, be sure to add the calories from your snack with the calories from your regular meals to obtain your correct daily total caloric intake. If in doubt, you can always ask your doctor about distributing your calories this way.

These slimming snacks are also permissible for those overweight persons who prefer the "nibbler's" approach instead of the regular Doctor's Special Menu Plan.

Perhaps you will like to eat a three-inch celery stalk, which is five calories. Chew it slowly and enjoy the crunchy sensation. This also adds bulk to your diet. A stalk of celery stuffed with cottage cheese and diced shrimp makes an attractive hors d'oeuvre.

The things that are impossible with men are possible with God.
—Luke 18:27

200-CALORIE SLIMMING SNACK SUGGESTIONS

	CALORIES
1 medium chicken thigh, broiled, skin removed	150
½ cup skim milk or non-fat buttermilk	40
	190
2 oz. roasted turkey	130
1 oz. skim-milk cheese	100
	230
2 oz. cold roast beef	180
½ cup skim milk or non-fat buttermilk	40
	220
1 oz. cold roast beef	90
1 oz. skim milk cheese	100
	190
2 oz. broiled beef patty	130
1 hard-boiled egg	75
	205
2 oz. water-packed tuna	90
1 oz. skim-milk cheese	100
	190
1 all-beef frankfurter	110
1 cup skim milk or non-fat buttermilk	85
	195
2 oz. chicken livers	80
1 oz. skim-milk cheese	100
½ cup skim milk or non-fat buttermilk	40
	220
2 oz. broiled beef patty	130
1 cup skim milk or nonfat buttermilk	85
	215

3 oz. canned salmon	120
1 cup skim milk or nonfat buttermilk	85
	205

2 oz. broiled beef patty	130
4 Tbsp. low-fat cottage cheese mixed with the patty	40
	170

3 oz. dried beef	165
2 Tbsp. low-fat cottage cheese	20
	185

3 oz. water-packed tuna	130
1 hard-boiled egg	75
	205

1 hard-boiled egg	75
1 tsp. bacon substitute	45
1 cup skim milk or nonfat buttermilk	85
	205

½ cup low-fat cottage cheese sprinkled with	105
2 tsp. vegetable-type bacon	90
	195

½ cup low-fat cottage cheese	105
1 hard-boiled egg	75
	180

1 all-beef frankfurter	110
1 oz. skim-milk cheese	100
	210

3 oz. boiled shrimp	70
1 hard-boiled egg	75
½ cup skim milk or nonfat buttermilk	40
	185

3 oz. boiled shrimp	70
½ cup low-fat cottage cheese	75
½ cup skim milk or nonfat buttermilk	40
	215

2 oz. water-packed tuna	90
1 hard-boiled egg	75
1 cup bouillon	5
	170

1 slice all-beef bologna	95
1 oz. skim-milk cheese	100
	195

3 oz. chicken livers	115
1 cup skim milk or nonfat buttermilk	85
	200

3 oz. canned sardines, natural-packed	180
½ cup skim milk or nonfat buttermilk	40
	220

½ cup low-fat cottage cheese	105
1 slice all-beef bologna	70
1 cup beef bouillon	5
	180

Keep your mouth closed and you'll stay out of trouble.

—*Proverbs 21:23*

100-CALORIE SNACKS
SLIMMING SNACK SUGGESTIONS

	CALORIES
1½ oz. turkey, roasted	95
4 oz. boiled shrimp	94
3 oz. canned salmon	120
2 oz. water-packed tuna	43
½ cup skim milk	75
1 hard-boiled egg	118
3 oz. chicken livers, boiled	115
2 oz. broiled beef patty	126
2 oz. dried beef	110
2 oz. roasted chicken	110
1 all-beef frankfurter	110
½ cup low-fat cottage cheese	103
1 cup skim milk	85
1 cup buttermilk	85
1 cup low-fat yogurt	110
2 oz. lean corned beef	100
1½ oz. baked ham	93
1½ oz. beef liver	85
3 oz. pork liver	105
1 oz. dry-roasted peanuts	100
4 oz. broiled lobster	90
3 oz. cooked or canned crab	85
4 oz. steamed white bass	115
3½ oz. broiled trout	115
3 oz. boiled shrimp and ½ cup skim buttermilk	113
½ oz. dry-roasted mixed nuts	80
¼ oz. dry-roasted soy nuts	97

Do not eat the dry-roasted nuts often, as they have a higher percentage of fat calories than the other snacks.

6

YOUR FRIENDS
How to know allowable foods and their caloric content

ぷつぐ

- Beverages
- Breads
- Cheeses and eggs
- Fruits and berries
- Meats and fowl
- Seafoods and fish
- Soups
- Vegetables
- Miscellaneous

APPROXIMATE CALORIC VALUE OF ALLOWABLE (FRIENDLY) FOODS ON YOUR DOCTOR'S SPECIAL 500 - 1000 CALORIE DIET

Remember, low-calorie, low-fat, low-carbohydrate and high-protein foods are your friendly helpers in attaining and retaining a slim, healthy body.

BEVERAGES

		CALORIES
Buttermilk, nonfat	1 cup	85
Lemon juice	1 Tbsp.	5
Lime juice	1 Tbsp.	5
Milk, skim	1 cup	85
Milk, skim (powdered)	1 Tbsp.	25
Sauerkraut juice	½ cup	5
Tomato juice	1 cup	60
Vegetable juice (such as V-8)	1 cup	90
Carrot juice	1 cup	60
Club soda	8 oz.	5

BREAD PRODUCTS

Toast, melba	1 large slice	40
Tortilla	one, 5" diameter	55
Rye-Krisp	1 cracker	20
Zweiback	1 slice	30

CHEESES AND EGGS

Cottage cheese, low-fat	½ cup	105
Skim-milk cheese	1 oz.	60
Egg white	1 white	15

FRUITS & BERRIES

Apple, raw	1 med.	80
Apricots, raw	3 med.	60
Cantaloupe, one-half	5" diameter	45
Grapefruit, one-half	5" diameter	110
Honeydew melon	1 wedge—2"x7"	55
Lemon	1 med.	25
Lime	1 med.	25
Nectarines	1 med.	85
Orange	1 med.	80
Peaches, raw	1 cup, sliced	85
Plums, raw	1 med.	30
Tangerines	1 med.	105
Watermelons	½ slice, ¾"	50
Blackberries	1 cup	85
Blueberries	1 cup	90
Strawberries	1 cup	60

Dietetic canned fruit, water-packed or noncaloric sweetened:

Applesauce	½ cup	50
Apricot	2 halves	20
Fruit cocktail	½ cup	35
Grapefruit sections	½ cup	35
Peaches	½ cup	35

MEATS AND FOWL

Beef, dried or chipped	3 oz.	165
Beef, lean ground	3 oz.	190
Beef, heart	3 oz.	90
Beef, chuck	3 oz.	260
Beef, round steak	3 oz.	190
Beef, sirloin	3 oz.	250
Beef, tenderloin	3 oz.	225
Beef, tongue	3 oz.	170
Beef, liver	3 oz.	170
All-beef frank	1	110

Beef bologna	1 slice, 4½"x1/8"	70
Vegetable-type bacon	2 tsp.	90
Chicken, fryer, broiled	1 breast	200
Chicken, fryer, broiled	1 thigh	150
Chicken, heart	3 oz.	120
Chicken, livers	3 oz.	115
Frog legs	4 oz.	75
Rabbit	3 oz.	150
Turkey	3 oz.	190
Veal Cutlet	3 oz.	175
Venison	3 oz.	200

SEAFOODS

Abalone	6" fillet	75
Bass, white, steamed	4 oz.	115
Clams, canned or cooked	6 med.	45
Crab, canned or cooked	3 oz.	85
Lobster, canned	3 oz.	75
Lobster, boiled	4 oz.	90
Salmon, canned, pink	3 oz.	120
Salmon, fresh	3 oz.	100
Scallops, steamed	3 oz.	95
Shrimp, dry-packed	3 oz.	100
Shrimp, fresh	3 oz.	70
Trout	7 oz.	225
Tuna, water-packed	3 oz.	130
Whitefish	3 oz.	90

SOUPS

Bouillon	1 cube	5
Bouillon, canned	1 cup	30
Chicken, clear	1 cup	80
Consomme	1 cup	35

VEGETABLES

Artichoke	1 med.	15
Asparagus, canned	6 tips	30

Asparagus, fresh, cooked	6 tips	15
Beans, green or wax	1 cup	25
Beans, string	1 cup	30
Beans, soy sprouts	1 cup	60
Beet greens	1 cup	45
Broccoli	1 cup	50
Brussel sprouts	1 cup	65
Cabbage, boiled	1 cup	50
Cabbage, Chinese cooked	1 cup	35
Cabbage, raw	1 cup	25
Carrots, cooked	1 cup	45
Carrots, raw	1 cup	50
Cauliflower, cooked	1 cup	35
Cauliflower, raw	1 cup	30
Celery, cooked	1 cup	30
Celery, raw, diced	1 cup	20
Chicory	¼ head	10
Chives	1 cup	50
Cucumbers, raw	1 med.	25
Dandelion greens	1 cup	95
Eggplant	1 cup	25
Kale	1 cup	50
Kohlrabi	1 cup	50
Lettuce	¼ of l lb. head	20
Lettuce, Romaine	5 large leaves	10
Mushrooms	½ cup	25
Mustard greens	1 cup	40
Okra	8 med. pods	30
Onions, raw	1 Tbsp.	5
Onions, cooked	½ cup	45
Onions, young green	3	10
Parsley, raw, chopped	1 Tbsp.	—
Pepper, green, raw or cooked	1 med.	20
Radishes	4 small	5
Salsify (oyster plant)	½ cup	35
Sauerkraut, canned	1 cup	45
Spinach, cooked	1 cup	35
Squash, soft shell	1 cup	40
Swiss chard	1 cup	30

126
MISCELLANEOUS

Tomatoes, canned	1 cup	55
Tomato, raw	1 med.	55
Turnips	1 cup	45
Turnip greens	1 cup	50
Horseradish	2 tsp.	5
Pickles, dill	1 large	20
Pickles, sour	1 large	15
Pimento	1 tsp.	5
Vinegar	1 Tbsp.	5
Wheat germ	2 Tbsp.	30
Brewer's yeast	1 Tbsp.	30
Yogurt, nonfat	2 Tbsp.	20
Gelatin, unflavored	1 envelope	30

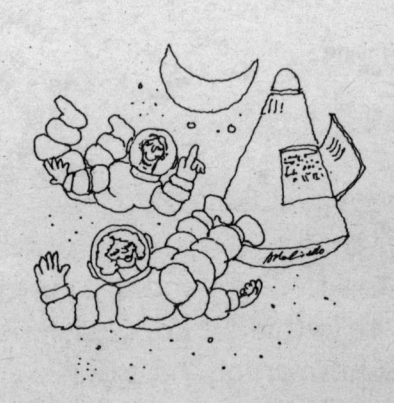

No wonder so many people want to be traveling in outer space—just to feel weightless.

7

NO LONGER HO HUM

Add glamor
while subtracting pounds
whether at a party
or in your own home

- Slender socializing
- Making your kitchen dietetic
- Glamorizing and decaloring food
- Taking fat out of your food
- Outsmarting the scales

SLENDER SOCIALIZING

Be sure to become familiar with the size of food servings your menu plan allows. Study so you will know by memory the required portions of allowable foods.

Cafeterias offer a greater choice of foods, but the better restaurants are often very cooperative in preparing suitable low-calorie foods.

When at parties, make your hostess happy by taking a low-calorie tidbit, but pass up the dips, chips, pastries, and other high-calorie foods. When your well-meaning friends try to force forbidden foods on you, mumble something very medical about your heart, your arteries, your blood sugar, etc. If they insist, then say plaintively, "You don't want to make me sick, do you?" Good luck!

BREAKFAST

Vegetable cocktail or V-8, skim milk or buttermilk, sauerkraut juice, cantaloupe, honeydew melon, orange, apple, strawberries, peach, melba toast, Rye-Krisp, Zweibach, cottage cheese, ½ grapefruit, dietetic or water-packed fruit cup.

APPETIZERS AND SNACKS

Celery sticks, carrot sticks or curls, raw oysters, sliced orange, radishes, cantaloupe, honeydew melon, ½ grapefruit, dietetic or water-packed fruit cup, apple, peach, watermelon, plum, strawberries, blueberries, blackberries, applesauce (dietetic), tomato or vegetable juice cocktail, cottage cheese, smoked chicken or turkey.

SOUPS

Clear soup, consomme, bouillon (chicken, vegetable, beef), vegetable soup, clam broth.

MAIN COURSES

Broiled or baked allowable fish; boiled, baked, or broiled shellfish, such as shrimp, scallops, crab, lobster, oyster; roasted or baked chicken, turkey, beef, or veal; broiled beef, pork, or chicken liver; vegetable plate; fruit plate; cottage cheese, plain or with fruit. Avoid cream or butter sauces.

SANDWICHES

Eat only that half the bun or bread having the least grease, butter, or mayonnaise on it. Better yet, avoid entirely the overprocessed, devitalized white flour in the bread or bun by eating only the meat.

VEGETABLES

All cooked or raw vegetables on the allowable list.
Vegetables served without butter, oil or cream sauces, either in preparation or serving. Lemon juice enhances the flavor of all vegetables.

SALADS

All allowable vegetables or fruits with special or dietetic dressings. No salads are acceptable that contain 15% or 20% carbohydrate vegetables or fruits.

DESSERTS

Cantaloupe, honeydew, or watermelon; all allowable fresh or unsweetened frozen or canned fruit; gelatin desserts.

BEVERAGES

Tea or coffee (no cream or sugar), skim milk or buttermilk, bouillon, tomato or V-8 juice, Perrier water with a slice of lime. No hot chocolate or cocoa.

YOUR DIETETIC KITCHEN

Since you are serious about losing weight, we must make your kitchen help you. Dieting is mainly a matter of adjusting your eating habits to a new life plan, a better lifestyle. So show your self-control and set up your kitchen for smart eating.

A supply cabinet and at least a part of your refrigerator should be stocked and rearranged to reflect your new calorie-conscious approach to cooking. These are key factors in your success. If they do not contain low-calorie foods or their ingredients, you are not winning the battle of the bulge.

Be sure that you have certain basic equipment in your kitchen. They are the tools of your trade. You're trading ugly fat for vitality and health.

Teflon pans are necessary in order to prepare foods without frying. The extra fat calories in fried foods make it impossible for you to stay on this special 500- or 1000-calorie diet. A broiler is necessary for the same reason. An electric blender or food processor will allow you to make many appetizing dishes and will save you a lot of time.

Fat-burning meals are measured meals, so you will need measuring cups and spoons. Diet scales (or your postal scales) are a must in order to learn to recognize the weight of your allowed portions of calorie-wise foods.

There are many important and useful low-calorie utensils and gadgets, such as: a vegetable slicer, shredder, and grater; a food chopper; a pepper mill; a good eggbeater; individual casseroles and ramekins; shell servers; molds; meat thermometers; a good roaster and meat rack; melon baller; fluted knives; shears. Add any other items you think will help you decalorize your food while making your dishes more attractive.

GLAMORIZED AND DECALORIZED FOOD

The more you curb calories, the more important it is for you to make your food look appetizing and taste delicious. Serve your food portions on a small plate, like a salad plate. Then you will seem to have more on your plate although you have smaller servings.

Be sure always to add the little touches to your food and your drinks. Remember to add a slice of lemon to your glass of tea, or maybe a touch of ginger or mint.

And don't forget to add a spray of watercress or minced parsley, or else a slice of pimento or a dash of paprika to increase the eye appeal of your dishes and servings.

Serve your coffee or tea (without cream or sugar, of course) after your meal. Take your cup to the den or living room and make an occasion of it.

Lemon juice, vinegar, or low-calorie salad dressings should be used on your salads. No oil is allowable because of its fat content.

Drink water or fluids 15 to 20 minutes before you eat. This will keep your stomach feeling fuller when you do eat your meal.

Always chew your food slowly. Your food will be more flavorful and filling.

Allow some elapsed time between the food items on your menu plans. This makes a small diet meal more satisfying and it will seem like more food.

TAKING THE FAT OUT OF YOUR FOOD

Low-calorie cooking is an art you can easily acquire. It can give you a new look and a new lease on life.

Low-calorie cooking can make you slim, happy, and comfortable in your new, smaller-size clothes, and (with your doctor's help) it can make you HEALTHY.

Since your old cooking habits have overlooked low-calorie food preparation, you will need to change your cooking habits. We are all creatures of habit. So, even though it may not be easy, we must change to reap the rewards of low-calorie cooking.

You can change many of your favorite recipes to low-calorie counts. It's easy . . . you can even fool your friends!

You must avoid, like the plague, all high fat- and sugar-containing foods. They are concentrated sources of the calories that you must shun. Starches are restricted. High-protein food is stressed because it is the vital food of life. Proteins are needed for every cell, tissue, and organ in the human body. They are the building blocks of body chemistry. They will safeguard your health.

Sometimes the method of preparation of low-calorie foods can make them very high in caloric values. Unwise food preparation reduces nutritional quality and increases calories. NEVER FRY ANYTHING. Frequently check your calorie tables.

Lean meat preparation requires low temperatures. Meat will be less tough and will shrink less. Broil lean meat whenever possible. Always drain fat released during cooking. Roasting is another good way to prepare lean meat for streamliners. Boiling (or rather, simmering—temperature should be between 180 degrees and 210 degrees, which is just below the boiling point) is good for less tender cuts of meat. Some lean meats can be stewed, but the fat must be skimmed off for dieters. Fried and breaded meats have absolutely no place in the reducer's kitchen.

Poultry should be broiled or roasted to save calories. Frying is NOT acceptable, nor is stuffing. Remove skin and fat. Don't stuff the bird and your body.

Fish should be broiled or steamed. Don't add fat when broiling. If it appears dry, add a drop of vegetable oil to the tip of your finger and rub it on the fish. Cooking time must be watched carefully as fish cooks quickly and loses flavor when overcooked. Fish and seafood are good protein foods, lower in fats than most meats, loaded with minerals from the sea, and comfortably low in total calories. But you must skip the frying of fish and seafood. Cream or butter sauces add calories fast, too, so they are also No-No's.

Fruit should be eaten fresh and raw with the skin on. They can be mixed for a fruit cup and sweetened with a noncaloric sweetener. Buy fruits in proper season. They are cheaper, fresher, and more nutritious. Canned fruit must be water- packed or dietetic-packed. Carefully check the sugar content of any canned fruit. NO fruit juices are allowed on your 500-calorie diet.

Vegetables are a boon to low-calorie diets but require protective cooking. Most are low in calories, and they are both filling and high in vitamins and minerals. Some of the better features of vegetables are their variety and abundance. Buying fresh vegetables is important, because they are very perishable, especially the watery types like watercress and celery. It is false economy to buy bruised, limp, wilted, or overripe produce.

Proper cleaning is essential. Residual herbicides and pesticides can affect our body chemistry by settling in our fat deposits. Use plenty of water to wash vegetables and fruits. Do not tear or bruise leafy vegetables, as they lose water-soluble vitamins and minerals through the broken areas. Root vegetables are best cleaned with brushes that are not too stiff. Scraping is better than peeling off most root vegetables.

Cook vegetables whole rather than in pieces, because mineral and vitamin losses occur when more surface is exposed. Quick-cooked vegetables look good, taste good, and are better for you. Overcooking, a too-common practice, makes them look and taste less appetizing. Also, cook vegetables at the last minute before serving, to avoid taste and value loss.

Here are some pointers for cooking vegetables in the slimline kitchen:

1. Steaming, either in a pressure cooker or a steamer, is excellent for vegetables. The fiber is softened with less nutritional loss.
2. Use as little water as possible for simmering. Do not allow brisk boiling. Use the liquid that is left over for soup stock.
3. Avoid excessive stirring, as that exposes vegetables to the air, which destroys some vitamins.
4. Cook quickly and covered until tender. A moderate oven is best for baking or broiling certain vegetables.
5. Frozen vegetables should not be thawed. Conserve vitamins by plunging frozen vegetables into boiling water and then reducing water temperature. Freezing and canning vegetables offsets the transportation loss of vitamins in some vegetables.
6. Do not oversalt. Use spices and herbs for zestful seasoning.
7. Beware of baking soda. It is very destructive to vitamins.
8. Serve all the raw vegetables you can. You are getting all the available vitamins and minerals when you eat your vegetables raw.
9. DON'T FRY. This is a strict taboo in the weight-conscious, calorie-wise kitchen. Frying adds the villainous fat calories and it also destroys vitamins.

One of the secrets of success in the dietetic kitchen is good seasoning. Herbs, spices, and condiments have no calories whatever, and they will add new taste experiences to your food. They should be used with discretion. It is better to use too little of an herb or spice at first than to overpower your taste buds with too much. However, almost any dish will gain flavor by the judicious use of seasonings.

OUTSMARTING THE SCALES

Get acquainted with other persons who share your enthusiasm for using the 500-calorie or 1000-calorie diet. You can benefit from the psychological encouragement you give each other. You will learn new food facts from discussing low-calorie menus and recipes.

Ask your friends, your co-workers, and your family to assist you in obtaining your goal. They must know that you are sincere. They will be even more helpful once they see that you are determined to become healthier and more attractive. By the time you begin to show results, you will receive plenty of help and encouragement. Be careful of those who might be envious of your goals and your self-control. They will not be helpful and may even encourage you to eat forbidden foods. They are not your true friends.

Learn to think positively. Positive power will be in your grasp always if you think and keep repeating to yourself: "I think I can." Read the best-selling book *The Power of Positive Thinking* by Norman Vincent Peale. It will help you to realize and reinforce your affirmative power. Practice your relaxation and visualization ritual every morning and evening. Think of the person you want to be. Plan your complete objective. Then, at night, think of what you did that day toward the accomplishment of that goal. Also, recognize the areas in which you failed, and promise yourself that you will improve on the next day. Many times during the day close your eyes and visualize in your mind's eye the new slim, attractive you.

Ask the Creator's help to strengthen your self-control. Repeat your own favorite prayers for guidance and support. Concentrate on today. Remember that yesterday is gone and there is nothing you can do about it. Tomorrow is not here yet, so do not burden your mind with its problems. Today is the time for action.

If you are going to a dinner party or eating in a restaurant, you may want to eat one of the high-protein, low-calorie snacks at home before you go out. Never leave your house hungry when you go out to eat. If possible, warn your hostess that you are on a low-calorie dietary intake plan for health reasons.

If you like to nibble, chew a few celery leaves, watercress sprigs, or mushroom buttons. You may season them with garlic powder, celery salt, or other flavorful seasonings. If you are a sipper by habit, sip lemonade made with noncaloric sweetener and water or unsweetened club soda, or try Perrier water and a slice of lime.

Learn and practice being selfish. Think of yourself first when it comes to preparing meals in your home. Think of yourself when you decide on a restaurant. Give your health and your dietary intake top priority in your life and in your home.

Do not follow your friends on foolish faddish diets. You may lose some weight on the scales, but you will also lose your precious health. This rapid weight loss which you may experience is due to loss of water from the destruction of your vital tissues.

Plan your day ahead so it will be easy for you to stay on your low-calorie meal-preparation program. Think of all your daily activities that do not involve food. Take pleasure in what you are doing at all times.

Try to exercise every day. Walk around your neighborhood. Walk to the bank. Walk to the grocery store. Walk to the drugstore. Walk to visit your friends. Make it a habit to walk as much as possible. Whenever possible, climb the stairs instead of taking elevators. Join your "Y". Many of them have exercise classes. Swim. It is an excellent exercise. Some spas and health clubs have very good exercise programs and helpful exercise machines to keep your skin tone and your muscle tone in good condition while you lose pounds.

Serve yourself limited quantities of food. Eat less and change your life so that living is a pleasure. Remind yourself that obese people have no fun.

Do not eat standing up or when you are on the run. Be sure that you are comfortably seated, and that you have a pleasant atmosphere and a relaxed attitude.

Use a smaller plate. The smaller food portions that you have been weighing and measuring will look larger on a smaller plate. Chew your food carefully. Take smaller bites. Put your fork down between each bite. This will slow your eating, as well as give you more time to enjoy the flavor of your meal.

Don't eat in bed. Be careful about eating while watching TV. If an ad for food appears on your screen, turn off your set or use your remote control device to change to another channel temporarily. Don't let yourself be psyched by hard-sell ads for foolish foods, for fast foods, for fat-causing foods.

It is best to eat in the same place in the house, where conditions are the most pleasant. This is preferably the kitchen or dining room.

Close your eyes and think good thoughts while you are eating. Eat slowly. Chew your food well before you swallow it. While you are planning your menu and preparing your meals, think pleasant thoughts. Believe that dieting is a pleasure, and it will be—particularly when you begin to see the results of your effort to have a healthy and attractive body.

Leave some food on your plate. Remember, calories are the yardstick used to measure the energy in your food as well as the energy output of your body. You must learn the amounts of calories in the food and drink that you prepare and consume.

Don't make excuses to yourself. If you do weaken and break your diet routine at a dinner in a restaurant or at a party, return to your dietary plans immediately. Don't abandon your weight-loss goal. Don't apologize even to yourself. Tell yourself that from now on you WILL do better. Don't wring your hands and abandon your weight-loss program because you made one little boo-boo.

Remember, if you cheat on your menus or recipes, you are really cheating yourself and yourself only.

You will find that the secret is learning not only *what* to eat, but also what *not* to eat. Your menus can vary within the allowable food group, but you must not eat the forbidden foods. You may, if you wish, hold back part of your day's allowable calories for the evening if you are a bedtime snacker. However, be sure you total ALL your calories daily.

As you lose weight, begin looking at more youthful fashions. This will inspire you because you know these more fashionable clothes will be your reward.

Check with a fashion counselor at your favorite store. She will point out the tricks of dressing yourself to make you look slimmer. Look at yourself naked in a full length mirror often. Weigh only when your doctor advises. Don't expect a weight loss every day. Your weight will vary during each day and from day to day.

Put a penny in a piggy bank for each calorie that you did NOT eat each day. Then, use the money to splurge on a new, attractive figure. Start now, tomorrow is too late. If you take care of yourself today, it will be easier to take care of your tomorrows.

Don't be discouraged if weight correction seems slow sometimes. You *can* lose weight and you WILL—if you don't cheat on your calorie intake and if you consistently follow your doctor's advice.

Thine, O Lord, is the greatness and the power and the glory and the victory.

—Chronicles 29:11

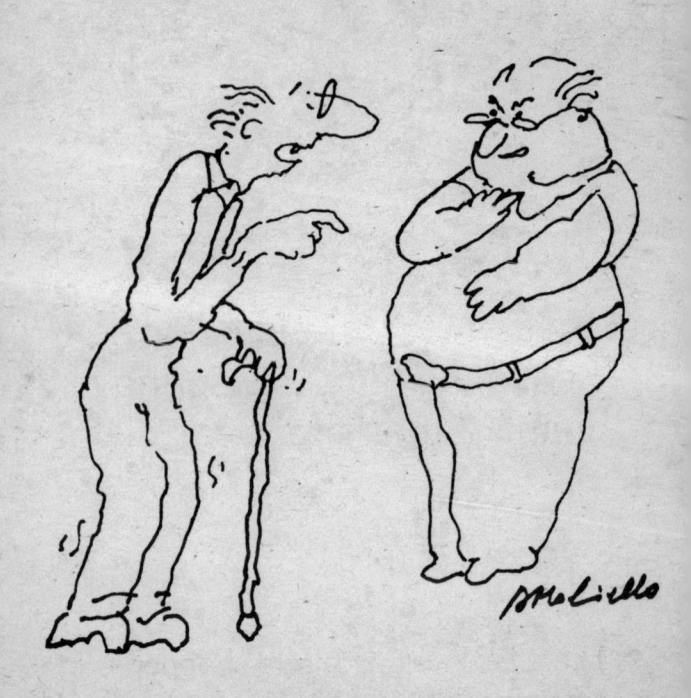

"A man is getting old when his chest and waist begin changing places."

8

MAKE IT EASY
The shopping, reading, counting, and measuring that are musts for your diet

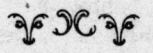

🙞 ❄ 🙜

- Hints for the low-calorie shopper
- Carbohydrate classification of fruits and vegetables
- Measurement tables

LOW-CALORIE SHOPPING HINTS

Your grocery store is the starting point for your low-calorie meals. By doing your marketing with extreme care you will find your job of food preparation much easier.

Check your weekly menus and the shopping list which precedes each section. Be sure you shop completely and thoroughly—extra trips to the store mean extra temptation. Many a weight-correction program has failed because the proper ingredients were not available and unpermitted items were substituted in preparation.

Do not shop when you are hungry!

Do shop when the store is not busy. Try a Monday or Tuesday—midafternoon if possible.

Explore the diet-food section of your supermarket . . . but BE CAREFUL. Many items which used to be available only in the diet-food section at a premium price are now available in the regular sections. Keep your eye out for water-packed fruits, tuna, and salmon, for example.

Be a label reader. Many items listed as "low-calorie" on the labels really aren't.

Hunt up a health-food store—you'll be surprised at the variety of dietetic items they carry. Also available are wheat germ and brewer's yeast, which can improve the nutritional quality of your low-calorie dishes and beverages. Remember to be a label reader —and don't let yourself be talked into inappropriate items. Let this book be your guide.

CLASSIFICATION OF VEGETABLES

Approximately 5% Carbohydrate

Artichoke
Asparagus
Beans, string
Beet greens
Broccoli
Cabbage
Cabbage, Chinese
Cauliflower
Celery
Chard
Collard greens
Cucumbers
Eggplant
Endive
Escarole
Kale
Leeks
Lettuce
Mushrooms
Mustard greens
Brussel sprouts
Pepper, green
Pickles
Pumpkin
Radishes
Rhubarb
Sauerkraut
Spinach
Squash, summer
Tomato or tomato juice
Turnip greens
Watercress

Approximately 10% Carbohydrate

Beets
Carrots
Celery root
Kohlrabi
Chicory
Chives
Dandelion greens
Onions
Peas, green
Pepper, red
Soybeans, fresh
Rutabaga
Squash, winter
Turnips

Approximately 15% Carbohydrate

Beans, dry
Beans, lima
Parsnips
Peas, black-eyed
Salsify
Soybeans, dry
Lentils

Approximately 40% Carbohydrate

Potato, sweet

CLASSIFICATION OF FRUITS

Approximately 5% Carbohydrate

Avocado (rich in fat)
Cantaloupe
Honeydew
Muskmelon
Watermelon

Approximately 10% Carbohydrate

Blackberries
Cranberries
Currants
Gooseberries
Grapefruit or
grapefruit juice
Lemon
Papaya
Strawberries
Tangerines

Approximately 15% Carbohydrate

Apple
Applesauce
Apricots, fresh
Blueberries
Grapes
Huckleberries
Kumquat
Lime
Loganberries
Mulberries
Nectarines
Oranges or orange juice
Peach
Pear
Pineapple/pineapple juice
Plums
Quince, fresh
Raspberries

Approximately 20% Carbohydrate

Banana
Cherries
Figs, fresh
Grape juice
Persimmon, Japanese
Prune juice, canned
Prunes, fresh

Above 20% Carbohydrate

Cherries, maraschino
Currants, dried
Dates, fresh, dried
Figs, dried
Persimmons, native, fresh
Prunes, dried
Raisins, dried

9

CONSUMING CALORIES

How and why
you burn calories

❦❧❦

- Calorie energy output
- Calories used per hour according to body weight
- Example: One woman's daily calorie expenditure

MEASUREMENTS

Dash	less than 1/8 teaspoon
3 teaspoons	1 tablespoon
4 tablespoons	¼ cup
5 tablespoons plus 1 teaspoon	⅓ cup
8 tablespoons plus 2 teaspoons	½ cup
10 tablespoons plus 2 teaspoons	⅔ cup
16 tablespoons	1 cup (8 oz.)
2 cups	1 pint (16 oz.)
4 cups	2 pints
2 pints	1 quart
4 quarts	1 gallon

Can Sizes:

8 oz.	1 cup
#1 Picnic	1¼ cup
#1	1½ cup
#300	2 cups
#303	2 cups
#2	2½ cups
#2½	3½ cups
#1 Square	1 pound

Many of us don't know what poor losers are until we start dieting.
—Tom LaMance

Living on a budget may be the same as living beyond your means except that you have a record of it.

CALORIE ENERGY OUTPUT

Your energy expenditure (calorie output) depends on the amount of exercise you get, your activities, your resting and sleeping hours, and the vigor and tension at which you go about your usual work.

Every weight-correction program must be based on the simple principle of *taking in fewer calories than are expended to use the body's stored fat deposits*. The body's extra fat must be used as energy. Don't try to overdo the exertion to burn calories too fast, as it is dangerous for overweight persons.

APPROXIMATE CALORIES USED PER HOUR, ACCORDING TO BODY WEIGHT

ACTIVITY	100 lbs.	120 lbs.	140 lbs.	160 lbs.	180 lbs.	200 lbs.
1. Sleeping	.45	.50	.65	.70	.80	.85
2. Awake but lying down	.50	.60	.70	.80	.80	1.00
3. Sitting quietly or eating	.65	.80	.90	1.05	1.15	1.30
4. Reading aloud, writing, standing, or sewing	.70	.85	.95	1.10	1.25	1.40
5. Dressing and undressing	.75	.90	1.05	1.20	1.35	1.50
6. Singing or cooking	.80	.95	1.10	1.25	1.40	1.60
7. Driving a car or typing rapidly	.90	1.10	1.25	1.45	1.65	1.80
8. Ironing, cooking, dishwashing, or dusting	.95	1.10	1.30	1.50	1.65	1.85
9. Light exercise, gardening	1.10	1.30	1.55	1.75	2.00	2.20
10. Walking slowly (2.6 mph)	1.30	1.55	1.80	2.10	2.35	2.60
11. Carpentry, mental work	1.55	1.90	2.20	2.50	2.80	3.10
12. "Active exercise"; i.e., bowling	1.90	2.25	2.65	3.00	3.40	3.75
13. Walking moderately fast (3.75 mph)	1.95	2.35	2.75	3.10	3.50	3.90

14. Walking downstairs	2.35	2.85	3.30	3.80	4.25	4.70
15. "Severe" exercise	2.90	3.50	4.10	4.65	5.25	5.95
16. Swimming	3.25	3.90	4.55	5.20	5.85	6.50
17. Running (5.4 mph)	3.70	4.45	5.20	5.90	6.65	7.40
18. "Very severe" exercise	3.90	4.70	5.45	6.25	7.00	7.80
19. Walking very, very fast (5.3 mph)	4.20	5.05	5.90	6.75	7.60	8.45
20. Walking upstairs	7.20	8.60	10.05	11.50	12.90	14.35

EXAMPLE
100-Pound Woman's Caloric Expenditure

Activity	Body Weight		Calories Per lb.		Time	Total Calories Used
Sleeping	100	X	.45	X	8 hrs.	360
Housekeeping	100	X	.95	X	8 hrs.	760
Grooming	100	X	.75	X	1 hr.	75
Reading	100	X	.70	X	1 hr.	70
Watching TV	100	X	.65	X	2 hrs.	130
Meal activity	100	X	.65	X	1 hr.	65
Driving car	100	X	.85	X	1 hr.	85
Light exercise	100	X	1.10	X	2 hrs.	220

DAILY TOTAL = 1,765

Computing your energy output in calories expended daily for several days will give you a better insight into the calories needed to attain and maintain a healthful weight.

Weight control is no longer a vanity reserved for the weaker sex; today it has become one of the greatest health protective measures.

10

WHY EXERCISE
How to get started on sensible exercises

༡༢༡

- Beginning exercises
- Exercise instructions and illustrations

EXERCISE

Exercise reduces bulges by toning muscles. Exercise keeps you from getting flabby while you shed pounds on your 500-calorie or 1000-calorie diet.

Exercise, even if it is strenuous, does not burn up enough stored fat to cause you to notice a rapid weight loss on the scales. (Instead, it is the abrupt loss of fluids that is reflected in a rapid weight loss). However, exercise will firm you, tone your muscles, improve circulation, redistribute your weight, and improve your shape to better proportions. It will also produce a sense of euphoria or well-being.

Exercise should be done in moderation. It should be consistent. You should check with your doctor for instructions about progressing to more strenuous activities.

Exercise can only be truly beneficial when it is used in conjunction with proper medical treatment and a medically supervised, lowered caloric food intake. Exercise and medical care must be tailored to each individual's needs. Overexercising will tend to produce hunger pangs. Be prudent. Exercising beyond your reserves can be very harmful.

Study your energy caloric output chart. Try to increase your caloric output every day by increasing your activities and exercise. If you will increase your energy output by 500 calories every day, you will expend 3500 additional calories in just one week. This will mean that you have burned off approximately one additional pound of disfiguring fat deposits.

The following illustrated exercises are some tried-and-true movements which will begin to firm and tone most of the muscles of your body in a few minutes. They should be done daily, starting with a few of each exercise and building up gradually. Men can more rapidly increase the number of times these exercises are performed.

#1—Toe-Touching with Deep Breathing

Stand with feet far apart. Extend arms from shoulder level sideways.
(A) Bend forward, exhaling through your mouth slowly and completely. Touch right fingertips to left foot. Keep knees as straight as possible.

(B) Return to original position, then raise arms and lean backward as far as you can, while inhaling very deeply through your nose. Contract and pull in abdominal muscles. Maintain until you have to exhale.
(C) Bend forward, exhaling through the mouth very slowly, and touch left fingertips to right foot.
(D) Return to original position. Repeat abdominal muscle contraction and deep breathing.

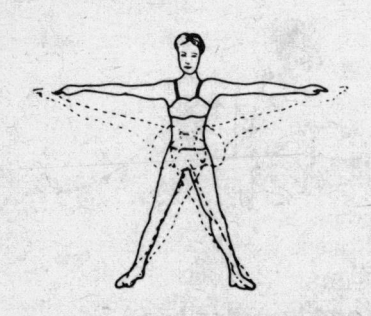

#2—Sit-Ups

Lie on back, flat on floor. Extend arms above head.
(A) Rise slowly to sitting position. Keep arms extended above head. Bend forward.
(B) Slowly return to original position, inhale deeply. Contract abdominal muscles. Maintain until you have to exhale.

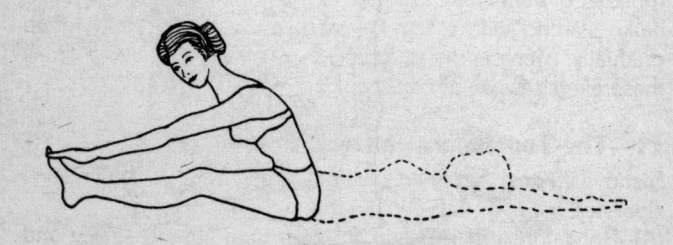

150
#3—Push-Ups
Lie on abdomen, hands below shoulders with palms down, weight on elbows.
(A) Straighten elbows and raise body off floor. Keep back straight and head elevated. Inhale deeply, contract abdominal muscles, maintain until you have to exhale.

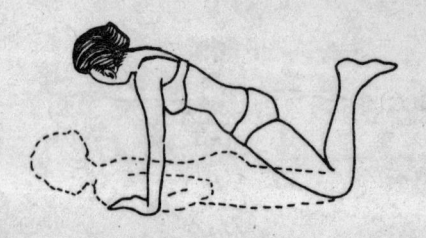

#4—Raising and Lowering Legs
Lie flat on floor on back. Hands at sides.
(A) Slowly raise both legs to perpendicular position.
(B) Slowly lower legs until feet nearly touch floor.
(C) Raise and lower legs several times until tired.

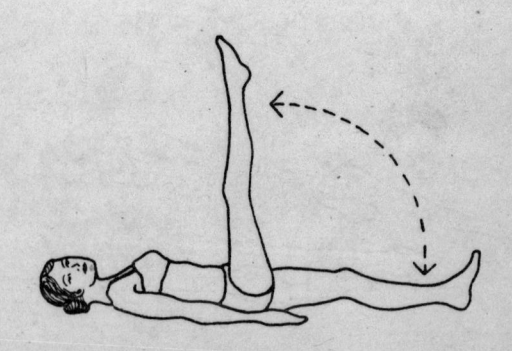

#5—Bicyling

Lie flat on floor on back, hands on hips. Raise hips, placing weight on elbows.
(A) Make full circles of bent legs in a bicycle-pedaling motion.

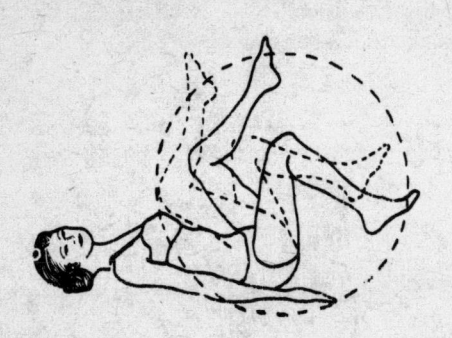

#6—Walking on Hips

Sit up straight, feet apart, knees straight. Extend arms forward at shoulder level.
(A) Shift weight onto left hip area. Pull right hip back while swinging both arms to the right and twisting the body to the right.
(B) Put weight onto right hip area. Pull left hip backward, swinging both arms to the left and twisting the body to the left.

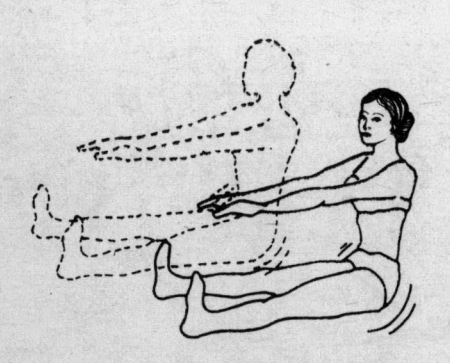

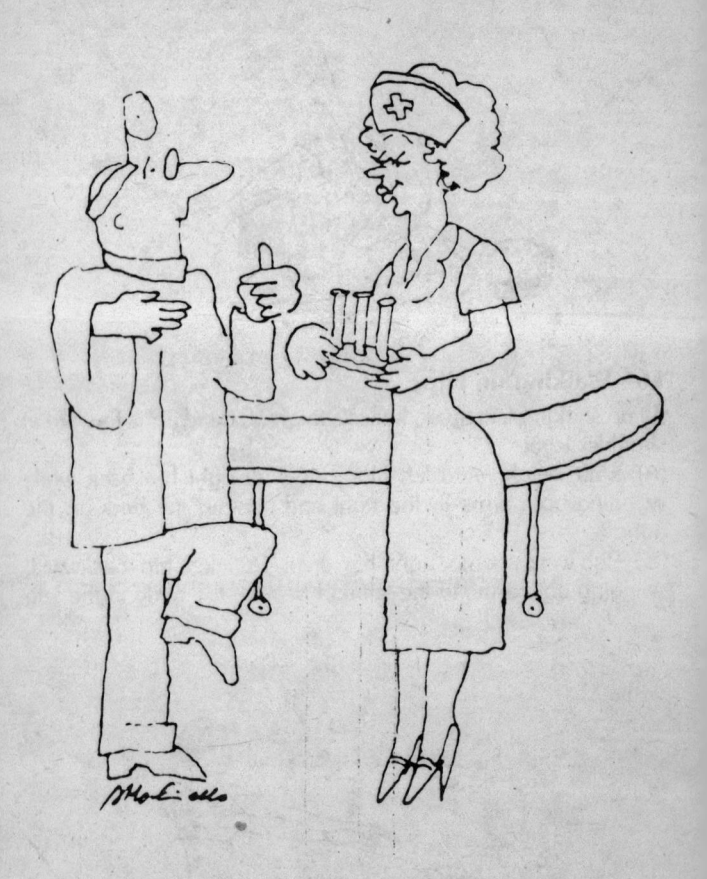

"One of my patients believes that a balanced diet is a milkshake in each hand."

11

THE ENEMY

Foods to avoid
and their caloric content

- Beverages and juices
- Breadstuffs
- Cakes, cookies, pies
- Cereals
- Cheeses and eggs
- Fats and oils
- Flour
- Fruits and berries
- Nuts
- Meats and fowl

BEVERAGES AND JUICES

		Total Calories
Apple juice	1 cup	130
Chocolate malt	1 cup	185
Chocolate milk	1 cup	195
Cocoa with milk	1 cup	250
Coconut milk	1 cup	65
Cola-type drink	1 cup	110
Ginger ale, dry	1 cup	80
Grapefruit juice, sweetened	1 cup	150
Grapefruit juice, unsweetened	1 cup	100
Grape juice	1 cup	175
Lemon juice, unsweetened	1 cup	75
Lime juice	1 cup	70
Milk, evaporated, canned	1 cup	175
Milk, whole or powdered	1 cup	170
Malted milk	1 cup	280
Milkshake, skim milk	1 cup	275
Orange juice, fresh	½ cup	60
Orange juice, canned, sweetened	1 cup	150
Orange juice, frozen, 6 oz.	1 cup	320
Pineapple juice, canned	1 cup	135
Prune juice, canned	1 cup	180
Root beer	1 small glass	45
Soda pop	1 small glass	40
Tangerine juice, canned or fresh	1 cup	105

BREADSTUFFS

Biscuit, baking powder	1 small	45
Bread, corn	2"x2"x¾"	80
Breadcrumbs	1 cup	330
Bread, Boston brown	1 slice	110
Bread, cracked wheat	1 slice	65
Bread, raisin	1 slice	65
Bread, rye	1 slice	60
Bread, whole wheat	1 slice	60

		Total Calories
Bread, white	1 slice	65
Cinnamon bun	1 slice	100
Crackers, graham	2 medium	55
Crackers, saltines	two, 2" square	30
Crackers, soda	two, 2½" square	45
Crackers, oyster	1 cup	60
Crackers, rye wafers	2	25
Macaroni, cooked	1 cup	210
Macaroni and cheese	1 cup	460
Muffins	1 2¾" diam.	130
Noodles, cooked	1 cup	50
Pancakes, wheat	one, 4"	60
Pancakes, buckwheat	one, 4"	45
Popovers	1	110
Pretzels	5 small sticks	10
Rolls	1	115
Rolls, sweet	1	180
Spaghetti, cooked	1 cup	215
Toast	Same caloric value as bread untoasted.	
Toast, cinnamon	1 slice	190
Toast, French	1 slice	110
Tortilla	one, 5" diam.	50
Waffle	one, 4½"x5½"x½"	210

CAKES

Angel food, plain	8", 2" wedge	110
Buckwheat cake	one, 4" diam.	45
Coffee cake	small	250
Chocolate layer	9", 1" wedge	110
Cupcake, plain	one, 2¾" wedge	130
Devil's food	9", 2" wedge	400
Coconut cake	1	140
Doughnut, raised	1	200

		Total Calories
Foundation cake	10", 1¼", 16th of 10" diam.	415
Fruitcake	12"x2"x½"	110
Gingerbread	½" cube	180
Jelly roll	½ slice	195
Pancake	one, 4"	60
Plain cake	one, 3"x2"x½"	180
Pound cake	one, 2¾"x3"x5/8"	130
Rich cake	one, 3"x3"x2"	115
Sponge cake	8" plain, 2" wedge	125
Strawberry shortcake	small serving 5½"	320
Waffle	one, 4½"x5½"x½"	210
Waffle with syrup	one, 4½"x5½"x½"	260

ICINGS

Chocolate	1 tablespoon	110
White	1 tablespoon	100

COOKIES

Chocolate	1	65
Cookies, plain	one, 3" diam.	110
Fig bar	1 small	60
Gingersnap	1	20
Macaroon, coconut	1	45
Molasses	1	35
Sugar	1	55
Wafer, plain	two, 2-1/8" diam.	45
Apple	9", 4" wedge	335
Apricot	9", 4" wedge	345
Blueberry	9", 4" wedge	290
Cherry	9", 4" wedge	380
Chocolate	9", 4" wedge	460
Coconut custard	9", 4" wedge	265
Custard	9", 4" wedge	265
Huckleberry	9", 4" wedge	295
Lemon meringue	9", 4" wedge	305

		Total Calories
Mince	9", 4" wedge	345
Peach	9", 4" wedge	340
Pumpkin, plain	9", 4" wedge	270
Pumpkin, chiffon	9", 4" wedge	415
Raisin	9", 4" wedge	395
Single	9" crust	655
Double	9" crust	1300

CEREALS

Bran flakes, all bran	1 cup	150
Bran flakes, 40 percent bran	1 cup	120
Bran, raisin	1 cup	155
Corn flakes	1 cup	95
Corn grits	1 cup	120
Cream of Wheat, cooked	1 cup	135
Farina, cooked	1 cup	100
Grapenuts	⅓ cup	55
Hominy, cooked	1 cup	115
Oatmeal, cooked	1 cup	75
Rice, cooked	1 cup	195
Rice flakes	1 cup	115
Rice, puffed	1 cup	55
Rice, wild, uncooked	1 cup	590
Special K	1 cup	85
Wheat flakes	1 cup	130
Wheat germ, stirred	1 cup	265
Wheat, puffed	1 cup	45
Wheat, shredded	¼"x2¼"	105

CHEESES AND EGGS

Blue	1 oz.	105
Camembert	1 oz.	85
Cheddar	1 oz.	110
Cheese souffle	1 cup	105

		Total Calories
Cottage, from whole milk	1 cup	25
Edam	1 oz.	10
Gorgonzola	1 oz.	10
Leiderkranz	1 oz.	8
Muenster	1 oz.	11
Parmesan, grated	2 teaspoons	2
Philadelphia cream	1 oz.	10
1 small package cheese	3 oz.	32
Pimento cheese spread	1 oz.	10
Processed cheese	1 oz.	10
Roquefort	1 oz.	10
Swiss	1 slice, 1 oz.	10

EGGS

*Eggs: whole, poached broiled, shirred	1 medium	7
*Egg yolk	1 medium	6
Egg omelet	2 medium	20
Eggs, scrambled	2 medium	20
Eggs, fried with pat of butter	2 medium	24

FATS AND OILS

Bacon fat	1 tablespoon	10
Butter	1 tablespoon	10
Butter	1 pat	5
Butter	1 cup	161
Cream, light, sweet or sour	1 tablespoon	3
Cream, heavy sweet or sour	1 tablespoon	5
Cod liver oil	1 tablespoon	12
Corn oil	1 tablespoon	12
Cottonseed oil	1 tablespoon	12
Crisco	1 tablespoon	12
Lard	1 tablespoon	12

		Total Calories
Lard	1 cup	1980
Margarine	1 tablespoon	100
Margarine	1 pat	50
Margarine	1 cup	1640
Mineral oil—no caloric value		
Olive oil	1 tablespoon	125
Olive oil	1 cup	1950
Peanut oil	1 tablespoon	125
Soybean oil	1 tablespoon	125
Suet	1 cup	800
Vegetable shortening	1 tablespoon	125

FLOUR

Corn, sifted	1 cup	400
Pastry, sifted	1 cup	375
Rye, sifted	1 cup	290
Soybean, stirred	1 cup	425
Wheat, self-rising, sifted	1 cup	385
Whole wheat, sifted	1 cup	400

FRUITS

Apple, baked	1 medium	200
Apples, cooked, sweetened	1 cup	310
Apple butter	1 tablespoon	35
Applesauce	1 cup	205
Apricots, water-packed	1 cup	80
Apricots, canned in syrup	1 cup	220
Apricots, dried, cooked and sweetened	1 cup	420
Avocado	one-half, 4" long	295
Banana	one, 6"x1½"	50
Cherries, fresh raw	1 cup	75
Cherries, canned	1 cup	140
Cranberries, raw	1 cup	60
Cranberry sauce, cooked	1 cup	560

		Total Calories
Currants, raw	1 cup	65
Dates, pitted	1 cup	510
Dates, plain	3 medium	80
Figs, fresh	three, 1½" diam.	105
Fruit cocktail	1 cup	190
Grapefruit, canned in syrup	1 cup	200
Grapes, raw slip skin Concord, etc.	1 cup	95
Grapes, raw adherent skin, Muscat, Thompson seedless, Tokay, etc.	1 cup	115
Guava, raw	1 medium	55
Mangos, raw	1 medium	100
Olives, green	10	75
Olives, ripe	10	115
Papaya, raw	1 cup	80
Peaches, canned	1 cup	195
Pears, fresh	1 cup	130
Pears, canned	1 cup	195
Persimmon, raw	one, 2¼" diam.	85
Pineapple, raw	1 slice	50
Pineapple, canned in syrup	1 slice	100
Plums, canned in syrup	1 cup	195
Prune, canned	3 medium	100
Prunes, cooked with sugar	1 cup	515
Prunes, cooked, no sugar	1 cup	305
Raisins, dried	1 cup	465
Rhubarb, cooked with sugar	1 cup	400
Watermelon	½ slice, ¾"	50

BERRIES

Cranberries, raw	1 cup	55
Cranberry sauce	1 cup	560

161
Total Calories

Currants	1 cup	65
Gooseberries	1 cup	70
Huckleberries	1 cup	90
Loganberries	1 cup	105
Raspberries, black	1 cup	110
Raspberries, red	1 cup	40

NUTS

Almonds	10	90
Almonds, shelled	1 cup	915
Brazil	3	130
Brazil, shelled	1 cup	970
Cashew, roasted	1 oz.	95
Chestnuts	5	65
Coconut, shredded	1 cup	360
Filberts, hazel	10	90
Peanuts, chopped	1 tablespoon	60
Peanuts, halved	1 cup	860
Peanuts, roasted	1 oz.	100
Pecans, chopped	1 tablespoon	60
Pecans, halved	1 cup	815
Walnuts, chopped	1 tablespoon	55
Walnuts, halved	1 cup	700

MEATS AND FOWL

Bacon, broiled, crisp	2 slices	95
Bacon, Canadian	4 oz.	250
Beef, boiled	4 oz.	235
Beef, chuck	3 oz.	260
Beef, flank	3 oz.	265
Beef, porterhouse	3 oz.	280
Beef, rump	3 oz.	310
Beef, stew	1 cup	295
Bologna	1 piece, 1"x1½" diam.	450
Brains	3 oz.	100

		Total Calories
Chicken, broiled	½, lean	320
Chicken, roasted	4 oz.	220
Chicken, stewed hen	4 oz.	330
Chicken, fryer, broiled	1 thigh	150
Chicken, creamed, a la king	1 cup	470
Duck, lean roasted portion	4 oz.	165
Frankfurter	1 average	125
Goose, lean roasted portion	4 oz.	150
Ham, cooked	3 oz.	330
Ham, boiled	3 oz.	250
Ham, canned, spiced	3 oz.	235
Ham, deviled	1 tablespoon	75
Hash, corned beef	3 oz.	115
Lamb chops, rib, med. fat	3 oz.	350
Lamb, leg of, roasted	3 oz.	220
Lamb, shoulder, roasted	3 oz.	285
Meat loaf, beef & pork	2 oz.	150
*Meat loaf, beef & pork	1 average slice	270
Mutton—see "lamb"		
Pork chop, broiled lean meat	1 average	285
Pork, ribs, roasted	3 ribs	125
Pork, loin roast	3 oz.	280
Pork sausage, link or bulk	4 oz.	500
Sweetbreads, boiled	3 oz.	160
Veal, leg, roast	3 oz.	210
Veal stew	3 oz.	240
Venison, broiled	3 oz.	200

SEAFOODS AND FISH

Bass, black, baked	4 oz.	230
Bluefish, broiled	4 oz.	180
Carp, broiled	4 oz.	130

		Total Calories
Codfish balls	one, 2" diam.	95
Codfish, creamed	½ cup	150
Haddock, steamed	1 fillet	100
Halibut, broiled	1 fillet	220
Herring, pickled	1 fillet	215
Mackerel, canned	3 oz.	145
Mackerel, fresh, broiled	3 oz.	160
Oysters, raw	1 cup	90
Oyster stew, with milk	1 cup	260
Perch, fried	1 fillet	110
Roe, shad	¼ cup	90
Salmon, canned, red	3 oz.	145
Salmon, king or Chinook	3 oz.	165
Salmon loaf	3 oz.	240
Sardines, canned in oil	3 oz.	275
Sardines, canned in tomato sauce	3 oz.	180
Sardines, natural-packed	3 oz.	170
Sole, broiled	3 oz.	135
Swordfish, broiled	one, 3"x3"x½"	210
Tuna, canned in oil	3 oz.	240

SOUPS

Asparagus, cream of	1 cup	225
Barley	1 cup	115
Bean, Yankee	1 cup	200
Beef broth	1 cup	100
Celery, cream of	1 cup	220
Clam chowder	1 cup	90
Corn, cream of	1 cup	190
Lentil	1 cup	375
Mushroom, cream of	1 cup	200
Noodle	1 cup	115
Onion	1 cup	105
Oyster, with milk	1 cup	170
Rice	1 cup	115

		Total Calories
Split Pea	1 cup	145
Tomato, cream of	1 cup	230

SWEETS

Butterscotch	1 oz.	115
Caramels	1 oz.	125
Chocolate creams	1 oz.	120
Chocolate syrup	1 tablespoon	50
Chocolate, sweetened with milk & nuts	1 oz.	165
Chocolate fudge	1 oz.	120
Chocolate mint	1 wafer	35
Chocolate, Hershey	2 squares	100
Citron	1 oz.	90
Cocoa, dry	1 tablespoon	20
Corn syrup	1 tablespoon	60
Ginger root	1 oz.	100
Gum	1 stick	15
Gumdrop	one, 1½" diam.	35
Hard candy	average piece	30
Honey	1 tablespoon	65
Jam	1 tablespoon	50
Jelly beans	4	30
Maple sugar	1 tablespoon	50
Marmalade	1 tablespoon	55
Marshmallow	1 oz.	90
Milk chocolate	2 oz.	300
Molasses	1 tablespoon	50
Peanut brittle	1 oz.	130
Peel, lemon, orange or grapefruit	1 oz.	90
Powdered sugar	1 tablespoon	30
Powdered sugar, stirred	1 cup	495
Sugar, brown, firm	1 cup	815
Sugar, brown, firm	1 tablespoon	50
Sugar cube,	one, 1/8"x5/8"x1/8"	25

		Total Calories
Sugar, granulated	1 tablespoon	50
Sugar, granulated	1 teaspoon	15
Sugar, granulated	1 cup	770
Apple betty	1 cup	345
Butterscotch pudding	½ cup	180
Chocolate beverage with milk	1 cup	255
Custard pudding	½ cup	100
Dates, plain	½ cup	260
Dates, plain	3 medium	80
Figs, raw	3 small	105
Gelatine, Knox	1 envelope	30
Ice cream	2-oz. scoop	130
Ice cream cone, pastry only	1 cone	15
Ice cream soda, chocolate	1 glass	375
Ice cream soda, vanilla	1 glass	295
Ices & sherberts	1 small scoop	60
Jello desserts, no nuts	1 average serving	90
Malted milk, chocolate	1 glass	185
Malted milk, chocolate, with ice cream	1 glass	405
Malted milk, powdered	1 oz.	115
Plum pudding	1 cup	200
Prune whip	2 oz.	250
Rice pudding	½ cup	140
Strawberry shortcake	small serving	315
Tapioca, cooked	½ cup	80
Vanilla cornstarch pudding	1 cup	270

VEGETABLES

Avocado	½ med.	295
Beans, baked, no pork	1 cup	230
Beans, baked, with pork	1 cup	300
Beans, kidney	1 cup	115
Beans, lima	1 cup	85

		Total Calories
Beets, not buttered	1 cup	65
Collards, cooked	1 cup	95
Corn, white, or yellow	5" ear	95
Corn, canned	1 cup	85
Dock or sorrel, raw	1 cup	110
Endive, raw	1 pound	110
Escarole, raw	1 pound	110
Hominy	1 cup	115
Onions, cooked	1 cup	45
Parsnips, cooked	1 cup	95
Peas, green, cooked	1 cup	110
Peas, black-eyed, cooked	1 cup	155
Peas, canned	1 cup	75
Peas, creamed	1 cup	270
Potato, white, boiled	1 med., 2½" diam.	105
Potato, baked in jacket	2½" diam.	100
Potato, french fried	eight, 2"x½"x½"	165
Potato, raw, fried	1 cup	485
Potato, hash-brown	1 cup	470
Potato, mashed, milk added	1 cup	165
Potato chips	10 med.	110
Potato, sweet, boiled	one, 5"x2"x½"	180
Potato, sweet, candied	one, 3½"x2¼"	315
Pumpkin, canned	1 cup	85
Rhubarb, cooked	1 cup	400
Rice, brown	4 oz.	400
Squash, summer variety soft shell	1 cup	40
Squash, winter variety, boiled, hard shell	1 cup	115
Succotash, canned	1 cup	265
Tomato puree, canned	1 cup	100
Watercress, raw	1 pound	100

MISCELLANEOUS

| Anchovy paste | 1 teaspoon | 20 |

		Total Calories
Apple butter	1 tablespoon	35
Banana split	average comp.	375
Beef marrow	1 tablespoon	170
Catsup	1 tablespoon	20
Caviar	2 teaspoons	45
Chili con carne, without beans	1/3 cup	170
Chili sauce	1 tablespoon	15
Chocolate, baking, unsweetened	1 oz.	175
Chocolate, sweet	1 oz.	145
Chow mein	1 cup	255
Cornstarch	1 tablespoon	30
Cranberries, raw	1 cup	55
Cranberry sauce	1 cup	555
Croutons, fried	five 1-oz. cubes	120
Dressing, poultry	1/3 cup	165
Meat drippings	1 tablespoon	100
Eggnog, plain	1/2 cup	95
French dressing	1 tablespoon	60
Gravy	1 tablespoon	50
Gum	1 stick	15
Hard sauce	1 tablespoon	50
Herring, kippered	4 oz.	265
Herring, pickled	4 oz.	215
Herring, smoked	3 oz.	175
Hollandaise sauce	2 tablespoons	155
Lemon sauce	1 tablespoon	40
Mayonnaise	1 tablespoon	90
Mustard, prepared	1 teaspoon	—
Olives, green	10 large	75
Olives, ripe	10 large	120
Peanut butter	1 tablespoon	100
Pickles, bread & butter	1 cup	125
Popcorn, plain	1 cup	50
Potato chips	7 large, 3" diam.	110
Potato salad	1/2 cup	220
Pretzels	5 small sticks	15

		Total Calories
Roquefort dressing	1 tablespoon	120
Vinegar	1 cup	30
White sauce	1 cup	435
Yeast, compressed, baker's	1 oz.	25

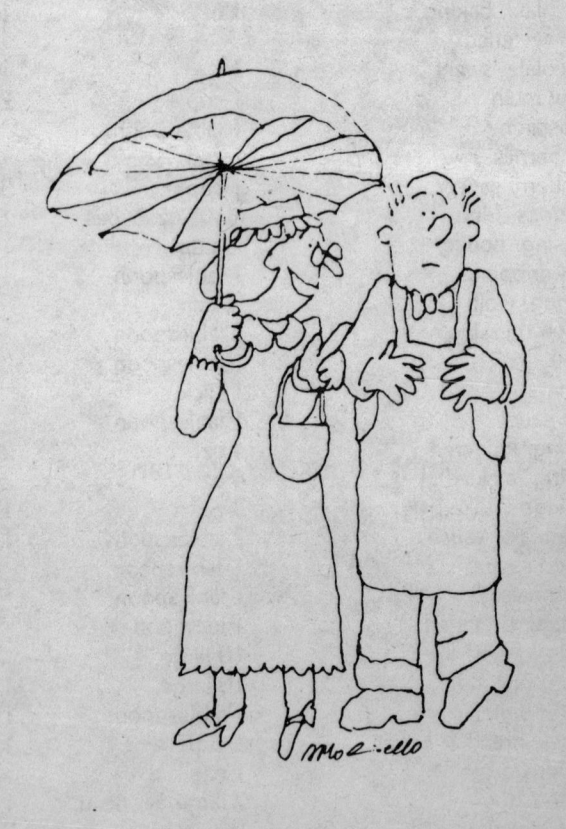

Middle age is when the torso becomes more-so.

12

MARKING PROGRESS
How to keep eat sheets and weight charts

☙❧☙

- Weight charts for women
- Weight charts for men
- Eat sheets

EAT SHEETS
YOUR DAILY CALORIC RECORD

MONDAY

	Food or Drink	Calories
Breakfast	_____	_____
Lunch	_____	_____
Dinner	_____	_____
Snacks	_____	_____
	Total	_____

TUESDAY

	Food or Drink	Calories
Breakfast	_____	_____
Lunch	_____	_____
Dinner	_____	_____
Snacks	_____	_____
	Total	_____

WEDNESDAY

	Food or Drink	Calories
Breakfast		
Lunch		
Dinner		
Snacks		
	Total	

THURSDAY

	Food or Drink	Calories
Breakfast		
Lunch		
Dinner		
Snacks		
	Total	

FRIDAY

	Food or Drink	Calories
Breakfast		
Lunch		
Dinner		
Snacks		
	Total	

SATURDAY

	Food or Drink	Calories
Breakfast		
Lunch		
Dinner		
Snacks		
	Total	

SUNDAY

	Food or Drink	Calories
Breakfast	_____	_____
	_____	_____
Lunch	_____	_____
	_____	_____
	_____	_____
Dinner	_____	_____
	_____	_____
Snacks	_____	_____
	_____	_____
	_____	_____
	Total	_____

WEIGHT CHARTS

These weight charts give the normal weight range for persons considered to be healthy. These are not average weights, which would mislead you, because most Americans tend to be overweight. These weight charts are compiled from various authoritative sources used by your doctor. Weight and height should be figured with shoes and normal clothes. What is YOUR desirable weight? Let your doctor make the final decision. He thinks of your health first.

WEIGHT CHART FOR WOMEN

Height	Small Frame	Medium Frame	Large Frame
4'10"	96-104	101-113	109-125
4'11"	99-107	104-116	112-128
5'0"	102-110	107-119	115-131
5'1"	105-113	110-122	118-134
5'2"	108-116	113-126	121-138
5'3"	111-119	116-130	125-142
5'4"	114-123	120-135	129-146
5'5"	118-127	124-139	133-150
5'6"	122-131	128-143	137-154
5'7"	126-135	132-147	141-158
5'8"	130-140	136-147	145-163
5'9"	134-144	140-155	149-168
5'10"	138-148	144-159	153-173
5'11"	142-152	148-163	157-177
6'0"	146-156	152-167	161-181

WEIGHT CHART FOR MEN

Height	Small Frame	Medium Frame	Large Frame
5'2"	115-123	121-133	129-144
5'3"	118-126	124-136	132-148
5'4"	121-129	127-139	135-152
5'5"	124-133	130-143	138-156
5'6"	128-137	134-147	142-161
5'7"	132-141	138-152	147-166
5'8"	136-145	142-156	151-170
5'9"	140-150	146-160	155-174
5'10"	144-154	150-165	159-179
5'11"	148-158	154-170	164-184
6'0"	152-162	158-175	168-189
6'1"	156-167	162-180	173-194
6'2"	160-171	167-185	178-199
6'3"	164-175	172-190	183-205
6'4"	168-179	177-195	188-210

NOTES